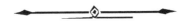

ISBN 978-0-364-44087-2
PIBN 10308139

Regional Anesthesia

(VICTOR PAUCHET'S TECHNIQUE)

BY

B. SHERWOOD-DUNN, M.D.

OFFICIER D'ACADEMIE; SURGEON (COLONEL) SERVICE DE SANTE MILITAIRE DE
PARIS; PHYSICIAN TO THE COCHIN HOSPITAL.

WITH 224 FIGURES IN THE TEXT

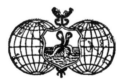

PHILADELPHIA

F. A. DAVIS COMPANY, PUBLISHERS

ENGLISH DEPOT
STANLEY PHILLIPS, LONDON

1920

PREFACE.

FOR thirty years Professor Reclus, of the Paris Faculté, preached and practised local anesthesia. His method consisted in infiltrating the tissues upon which he proposed to operate with a weak solution of cocaine—then proceeding with the operation.

This procedure is well known in France, and is often employed in minor operations.

Regional anesthesia differs widely from the method of Reclus. Instead of applying the anesthetic to the terminals of the nerves, it is injected at the point of the origin of the nerve, or along the trunk near the point of origin, so that the whole region supplied by the nerve and its branches is anesthetized. All the major as well as the most delicate minor operations can be performed in this way. The method has gained many adherents since 1914, and its growing popularity has led us to believe that an exposition of it would be welcomed by the American profession.

Professor Victor Pauchet is acknowledged to be the leading exponent of regional anesthesia in France, and this book constitutes a résumé of his writings upon this subject, together with those of P. Sourdat and J. Labouré. In addition there is included the latest experiences of Fauchet and the writer, together with Pauchet's recommendations, inserted during his revision and amplification of the manuscript before its transmission to the publishers.

I wish to acknowledge my indebtedness to Dr. Emilie Jané and Miss Frances Johnson, R. N., and to express my high appreciation of the assistance which they have rendered me in the preparation of this work for publication.

B. SHERWOOD-DUNN.

CONTENTS.

CHAPTER I.

CHAPTER II.

CHAPTER III.

CHAPTER IV,

CHAPTER V.

CHAPTER VI.

CHAPTER VII.

CHAPTER I.

GENERAL CONSIDERATIONS.

Advantages of Regional Anesthesia.

Anesthesia by injection possesses, as compared with anesthesia by general narcosis, advantages of such cardinal importance that, at the very outset, the reader's attention should be directed to them as ample justification for the time, labor and special education required to become sufficiently expert in its application to permit of its adoption for general employment.

Low Mortality Risks.—Since the concentrated solutions of cocaine have been replaced by weak solutions of the less toxic agents, such as stovaine, novocaine, procaine, etc., death from local or regional anesthesia has disappeared from surgical practice. The writer is unacquainted with a single case of death due to the employment of the last named anesthetics.

The relative rarity of death from narcosis (chloroform, 1 in 2000; ether, 1 in 5000) may make this advantage seem insignificant; but it is only necessary for an operator to lose one patient by narcosis, to have this apparently insignificant advantage brought forcibly to his attention.

(1)

Reduction of Post-operative Dangers.—General narcosis, aside from its mortality, produces complications which are of great importance because of their frequent occurrence. They include chiefly pulmonary complications, caused or aggravated by etherization, and alterations in the liver and kidneys through the action of ether, and particularly of chloroform. Rapid degeneration of the liver and kidneys following surgical operations is often attributed to shock or post-operative infection, but the fact that these accidents are eliminated by regional anesthesia would indicate that they are directly due to the action of the compounds used in general narcosis, and the superiority of regional anesthesia is made strikingly apparent in operations upon subjects suffering with chronic jaundice or renal insufficiency. The nausea and vomiting, which often continue for forty-eight hours after an operation and are such prominent factors in reducing the vital forces—especially in patients with strength already at the lowest ebb—are often the determining cause of death. These troublesome conditions are eliminated in regional anesthesia.

Diminution of Shock.—The reflex action of traumatism, the unconscious suffering of a patient even under the full influence of narcosis, is transmitted to the nerve centers, provoking disturbances which, repeated, result in certain alterations in the neurons, and these alterations constitute shock.

Local or regional anesthesia secures a complete physiological section of the nerves and suppresses completely this influence upon the nerve centers.

This fact has been so fully demonstrated that Crile (of Cleveland) practises local and regional anesthesia in all of his major operations, even when employing general narcosis with nitrous oxide. If comparison is made between a series of operations for cancer of the stomach under narcosis and a series under regional anesthesia, the relative condition of the patients subsequently offers a striking confirmation of the innocuousness of the latter procedure.

Absence of Danger from Asphyxia.—Administration of ether or chloroform is generally attended by greater or less respiratory disturbances. Onlookers often have their attention attracted by the patient's difficulty in breathing, due generally to mucus collecting in the mouth and nose, especially in the Trendelenburg position. Not infrequently the operator's attention is arrested by the same difficulty. All of this is absent in injection anesthesia.

Operations upon the respiratory tract, or in its vicinity, are greatly simplified and facilitated. The patient assumes whatever position is desired, being perfectly conscious. He can at will arrest his breathing, suppress a cough, or expectorate if need be. This is of valuable assistance in operations upon the pleura, larynx, neck, etc. In operations for goiter it safeguards the recurrent laryngeal nerve by allowing the patient to speak, thus calling attention to the nerve.

Special Advantages in Certain Operations.—
The fan-like distribution of the nerves after they
leave the large nerve trunks permits the performance of extensive operations once the trunk
has been anesthetized.   Thus a bronchial tumor,
or the cervical glands can be removed, or total
laryngectomy or external esophagotomy performed
after preliminary infiltration of the cervical plexus.

Nephrectomy can be painlessly performed after
paravertebral infiltration of six intercostal and
two lumbar trunks; not only are the parietes
rendered insensible, but the kidney can be sutured
or the pedicle liberated and ligated without pain.
The same advantage attaches in operations upon
the liver and stomach.   The rectum can be excised
after injecting through the sacral foramen.

Compared with the method of local infiltration,
practised by Reclus, regional anesthesia possesses
the following advantages:

(1) *The anesthesia is entirely distinct* from the
operation proper, being instituted beforehand, and if
possible, by an assistant in an adjoining room.   Consequently, successive operations can be performed
without loss of time.

(2) Once the nerve or nerves have been properly
anesthetized, the *anesthesia continues complete for
from one and one-half to two and one-half hours*
and the operation is never interrupted to make additional injections as is often the case in infiltration
anesthesia.

(3) It obviates all danger *of necrosis of the tissues,* such as sometimes occurs in local infiltration

where a section of the skin is mobilized in a plastic operation to cover a denuded surface and is nourished only by a narrow pedicle.

DISADVANTAGES OF REGIONAL ANESTHESIA.

Special Training Required.—Some training in the practical method of application is required to permit of successful practice of this procedure—though not more than is necessary for the execution of any of the simpler types of surgical operations.

As the simplest and most rapid procedure for securing the necessary experience we advise that the operator, after reading the detailed descriptions herein presented, first practise finding upon the skeleton, with needles of varying lengths, the cranial, spinal, intercostal and sacral nerve foramina.

When he has become familiar with the depths and directions of the various punctures through exercises upon the skeleton, the student of the method may then repeat the various operations upon the cadaver, using the longer and coarser needles and a fluid containing India ink. Dissection of the more difficult regions, after such experimentation, will disclose any faults and soon draw the operator's attention to any necessary corrections. Too much time need not be spent in this experimental work, however, before the operator begins upon the living subject, as no harm results from the injection of the fluid. But little actual experience is required for the surgeon to become confident and adept in finding the nerve trunks, this being facilitated by the more or less pronounced sensation referred to the terminal distributions when the point of the needle touches the nerve trunk, or by the insensibility of the surfaces supplied.

It will assist the operator in rapidly gaining confidence and skill if he will use at first a larger amount and a stronger solution and infiltrate a more extensive area.

Necessity of Gentleness and Skill in Operative Technique.—It is obvious that where an operation must be done ·with the complete consciousness and oftentimes in full view of the patient, a gentle, unhurried, and quiet technique is imperative and is conducive to a greater degree of satisfaction to the patient, with better results.

Some operators are accustomed to break up adhesions and carry out many surgical maneuvers with their hands and fingers. With injection anesthesia in abdominal operations especially, all pulling, tearing, and rough treatment should be avoided, as even with complete insensibility of the parts the patient cannot but be cognizant of the methods employed, and any such treatment produces an unfavorable mental impression which is prejudicial to final success. The scalpel and scissors should be used for all necessary separation of parts. Again, it is the habit of some to employ in their operations a variety of retractors, which are often the cause of unnecessary traumatism to the parts. This may also be said of the employment of an unnecessary number of pressure and rat-tooth forceps.

It must not be overlooked that a difference exists between sensation and pain; unnecessary pulling and handling of parts produces a disagreeable sensation which is likely to cause complaint on the part of the patient.

The more gently and quickly the operator proceeds, the greater will be his measure of operative success.

Objection that the Method Procures only a Partial Anesthesia.—In regional anesthesia it has been our experience that, out of 20 cases, 12 are completely insensible; 7 are sufficiently insensible to all necessary manipulations to permit of the operative procedure without serious complaint on the part of the patient; while 1 case out of 20 is found insufficiently anesthetized and must be given a little ethyl chloride to overcome the deficiency. Even in this event the quantity of inhalation anesthetic required is very slight.

The value of regional anesthesia is demonstrable by comparison, chiefly with general narcosis. The reader need only be reminded of the distressing experiences which attend the beginning and the close of the latter procedure, and but little experience with the former will convince any expert operator of its marked superiority. Apart from the distressing period of vomiting which follows general narcosis, the after pains complained of during the succeeding day and night are usually greatly diminished in regional anesthesia, and after nephrectomy, laparotomy, and facial operations a lasting condition of hypoanesthesia may often be noted, which renders the injection of morphine or other narcotic during the succeeding twenty-four hours unnecessary.

True, the patient will often complain at some time or other during the course of the operation. One says the table is too hard; another asks if the operation will not soon be finished; many complain of suffering because they confound sensation with pain. One of our patients cried out when he heard a fragment of his rib fall into the slop basin. These are minor inconveniences which it is well to be aware of in order to be prepared for them when they become manifest. The table should be well padded. In nervous and sensitive cases it is advisable to .blindfold the patient's eyes and to stop the ears with cotton.

Before all operations the patient should be given an injection of scopolamine-morphine, which not only does not interfere with, but rather assists the method. Absolute silence should be maintained in the operating room.

Necessarily the operator must have become perfected in the details and technique of the regional form of anesthesia. Any operator who, in the anesthetization of his patients, has had to rely upon the services of different assistants, knows how seldom a good one is found. The number of patients who are insufficiently or imperfectly brought under the anesthetic and bear down or resist during the course of the operation is legion, while not infrequently cases absorb too much of the anesthetic, causing the operator to discontinue his work while the patient is brought back from the danger line. It is not too much to ask, therefore, that the operator intending to make use of regional anesthesia should carefully and completely train himself in the details of the procedure and persevere in his technical practice until he has reached a satisfactory degree of perfection, just as he does in any and every other department of medical practice.

An important feature that should never be lost sight of is the psychology of the patient. Those who accept the method reluctantly, and are anxious, nervous, and hyper-sensitive, are the difficult subjects; most of these, however, once the operation has been satisfactorily concluded, express themselves as completely satisfied.

On the other hand, there are those who, familiar with the distress of the after-effects of general narcosis, welcome the new mode of procedure and make most satisfactory subjects. The mental attitude of the patient has almost as much to do with the success of the operation as the ability of the operator.

The Time Element.—About the same time is consumed in the administration of regional anesthesia as in that of general narcosis. About ten or fifteen minutes are required for an experienced assistant to perform the necessary injections in the former procedure, and another ten minutes must then elapse for the full effect to become established. About the same length of time is required to obtain the complete effects of inhalation anesthesia.

Where the operator is dealing with a private case, it is not often that a few moments more or less will particularly interfere with the type of technique he may select, that which is best in his opinion governing the choice.

In hospital service, where several cases are to be operated upon, it is essential to have an experienced assistant for the advance preparation of the cases. This likewise applies in the administration of a general anesthetic.

In any event, the loss of a few moments' time is not to be considered in comparison with the benefits to the patient that attend the regional form of anesthesia.

The Claim that Regional Anesthesia is not Equally Adapted for all Operations.—The beginner in regional anesthesia may better satisfy both himself and the patient by giving ethyl chloride, ether, or chloroform to complete the anesthesia if there is complaint to any degree.

Mixed anesthesias, although not attractive in theory, cause less shock than simple narcosis.

If a preparatory injection of morphine-scopolamine is administered before the introduction of the procaine-suprarenin and the operation is completed with the aid of the inhalation narcotics referred to, the patient will be affected less than by simple narcosis, *i.e.,* he will be less affected by three agents than by one. For this a theoretical explanation is available, but such explanation is not so important as the fact itself which has been learned by actual experience.

In trephining operations, goiter excisions, total laryngectomies, prostatectomies, operations for hemorrhoids, radical cure of hernia, and costal resections, regional anesthesia is a most gratifying procedure. With increasing experience, furthermore, the operator will learn the details of technique that render this form of anesthesia applicable to any and all operations.

CHAPTER II.

ARMAMENTARIUM.

Syringes.—The operator should have at his disposal Luer's all glass morphine syringe of 1- to 2- mil capacity, and also a metal and glass syringe of 10-mil capacity.

My earlier experience was with the Record syringe, which is very serviceable, but more lately I have been led to substitute the Collin all metal syringe (Fig. 1), which is to be preferred in that it is both short, powerful, and unbreakable. The syringe should be thoroughly water tight and provided at its top with lateral handles by means of which a firm hold can be secured.

Needles.—These should be of small caliber, with a short-beveled point. The smaller the caliber of the needle, the less painful its introduction. Needles of the smallest caliber and with long, fine points should be particularly employed for the formation of the dermal wheals later to be described.

Platinum needles are expensive and soon become blunted at the point. Steel needles are finer pointed and remain sharp longer, but are prone to rust and are easily broken. I have found it best to employ either fine steel, or nickel needles. The latter remain sharp and in good condition the longest. The junction between the nozzle of the

(12)

syringe and the needle must permit of no leakage, the needle remaining *in situ* while the syringe is repeatedly removed for refilling. The smooth

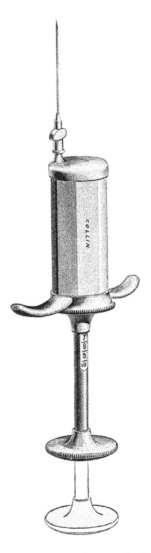

Fig. 1.—A 10-mil metal syringe of Collin make, short, strong, unbreakable, handy and with graduated plunger rod. The lateral socket enables the operator to make injections parallel with the surface while using a straight needle.

socket type should be chosen rather than the screw or bayonet form.

We employ only the straight form of needle. It is less expensive and more easily obtained, and when once one is accustomed to its use, it answers every purpose.

There should be provided needles of four lengths, viz., 3, 6, 9, and 12 centimeters (Fig. 2). The 3-centimeter needle is used in making the dermal wheals. It should be sharp pointed. The 12-centimeter needle is seldom used—chiefly for pre-sacral injections. The 6- and 9- centimeter needles serve for all general purposes.

To mark the exact depth to which the needle is to be introduced, the operator may make a shield from a piece of boiled cork or a square of rubber sheeting, to be adjusted upon the needle at the point desired.

The instruments and receptacles for the solution should be sterilized in plain boiling water, without addition of any chemical agent whatever.

Anesthetic.—As anesthetic we have been using *néocaïne-surrénine* (*Corbière*), a French preparation which replaces with perfect satisfaction the German product novocaine-adrenalin. In preparing a considerable amount of the solution, to be kept for some hours, it is best to use the pure procaine,[1] to which can be added immediately before use the required quantity of adrenin.

------

[1] Procaine being the term now in general use in the United States in place of neocaine or novocaine, this term will be regularly employed hereinafter.

The formulas of the mixtures used are as follows: (1) 25 drops of 1 to 1000 adrenin solution to 200 mils of ½ per cent. procaine solution;

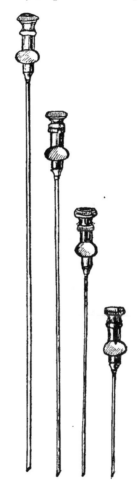

Fig. 2.—Four steel needles, respectively, 12, 9, 6, and 3 centimeters in length. Each needle is provided with a mandril. Actually the needles are twice as fine as they are represented in this illustration.

(2) 25 drops of adrenin to 100 mils of 1 per cent. procaine; (3) 25 drops of adrenin to 50 mils of 2 per cent. procaine; (4) 25 drops of adrenin

solution to 25 mils of 4 per cent. procaine. Twenty-five drops of the adrenin solution is the equivalent of 1 milligram of adrenin.

We use the 4 per cent. solution but seldom, for the cranial nerves and brachial plexus; the 2 per cent. solution frequently, as a rule for the nerve trunks; but the 1 per cent. and especially

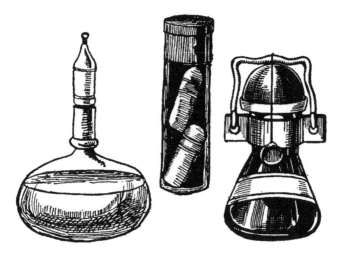

Fig. 3.—From left to right, an ampoule of saline solution for dissolving the procaine; a tube containing 2 capsules of procaine in powder form and 3 sealed flasks containing 150 grams of ½ per cent. solution.

the ½ per cent. solutions are those most commonly employed, the latter for all infiltrations.

It is far cheaper to prepare the solution as required than to buy it ready made.

The adrenin and procaine come in glass ampoules. On the evening of the day preceding the operation these are dissolved in boiled salt solution. Even more convenient are the procaine tablets which can be dissolved in boiled salt solution and kept until needed for use, when the required amount of adrenin is added.

It is inadvisable to attempt to sterilize the solution after the mixture has been made; this should be done beforehand. The procaine adrenin should be added to a hot solution (35° C.) to insure its ready dissolution.

The high percentage solutions should be injected very slowly, and in amounts never exceeding 20 to 40 mils of the ½ per cent. solution. We have employed, however, as much as 300 mils without any harmful effect.

In removal of the breast for cancer, as much as 250 to 300 mils may be employed; most of it escapes after the primary incision has been made.

For anesthetizing the viscera, and especially the peritoneal ligaments, the omental tissues, the meso-appendix, the mesentery, and the sero-vascular pedicles, we often employ (following the advice of Crile, of Cleveland) a 1 per cent. solution of quinine and urea hydrochloride,[1] injecting as much as 100 grams in addition to the solution of procaine-adrenin already used.

General Technique.

Theoretically, regional anesthesia and anesthesia by infiltration, according to the procedure of Reclus, are *two different methods*. Practically, neither of them excludes the other, but, in fact,

---

[1] The product termed by Corbière urocaïne.

they supplement each other and are often employed in combination.

The principle of regional anesthesia is, not to
infiltrate the field of operation or surrounding tissues, but to secure insensibility by directly injecting the nerves distributed to the region or tissues
surrounding these nerves. To each region corresponds a special technique, appropriate for the
insensibilization of the nerves in that region, and
with which the operator must be familiar in order
to succeed.

*Necessity of Perfect Asepsis in Regional Anes-
thesia.*—In making the injections, the operator
proceeds without gloves, but with hands well disinfected, as for an ordinary minor operation. The
instruments and solution must be sterilized. Care
is taken not to dip the syringe into the glass re-
ceptacle containing the solution, particularly if the
syringe has come in contact with the fingers of the
operator and the patient's skin. A special needle
is reserved for drawing up the fluid into the
syringe. It should be constantly borne in mind
that ungloved hands are never aseptic any more
than is the patient's skin.

In practice, the two methods, nerve-block-
ing and infiltration, are usually employed together,
the one aiding and completing the other.

With few exceptions, *e.g.*, anesthesia of the
meso-appendix with urocaine before its section, or
anesthesia of the omental tissues, complete induc-
tion of anesthesia precedes the operative procedure. No injection should be made during the

operation, which is performed as though the patient were under general anesthesia; the anesthesia should be complete when the patient is brought
to the surgeon, and there should be no more ques-
tion of it during the operation.

The method does not in any way prolong the
duration of the operation, nor does it leave the
operative field or the incision any longer exposed
to the air.

Preparation of the Field of Operation.—Before
the injections are begun, the skin of the field of

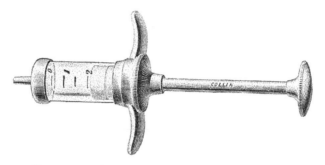

Fig. 4.—A 5-mil syringe of metal and glass.

operation should be disinfected with a 5 per cent.
tincture of iodine. When the injections have been
completed the region should be rubbed with alcohol, which will remove the few drops of liquid
injected and the excess of iodine. Next come the
final preparation of the patient, the covering of
the operative field, and the preparation of the
operator and his assistant—during which time the
tissues will have become completely anesthetized.

The Injections.—The syringe (Fig. 4) is held
with the thumb and the second and third fingers

of the right hand (Fig. 5). By virtue of the
flexibility of the operator's wrist, all pressure
other than that in the direct line of the needle
is obviated, to avoid breaking of the needle. The
latter should never be inserted down to its flange.

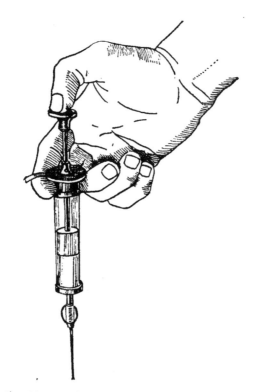

Fig. 5.—Shows the manner of holding the syringe
during injection. (*Reclus.*)

The plunger should be pushed home during the
introduction or the removal of the needle, the two
acts being simultaneous (*continuous injection of
Reclus*). The minimum quantity of ½ per cent.
solution to be injected is 1 mil per centimeter of
distance; for the 1 per cent. solution, slightly less.

The slight edema resulting from the subcutaneous injection raises the overlying skin, and the region injected, rendered ischemic by the adrenin, becomes definitely pale.

Difficulties arising from edema of the superficial tissues may be obviated by commencing with deep injections.

Skin Wheals.—In infiltrating a given region, it is· often necessary to make successive injections

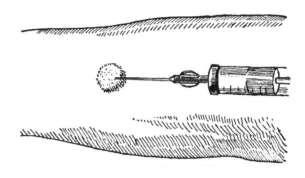

Fig. 6.—Formation of the dermal wheal. (*Pauchet.*) The bevel of the needle point is directed upward and should disappear entirely in the dermis before the intradermal injection is made.

with needles chosen progressively longer. Again it is indispensable to mark beforehand the sites for these injections by the formation of *"intradermal wheals"* which will render the skin insensitive to the introduction of the needle. The ·wheal consists essentially of an intradermal infiltration of small diameter (Fig. 6).

A fine, short needle mounted on a syringe filled with ½ per cent. solution is introduced almost parallel with the skin surface, with the bevelled edge upward, directly into the thickness of the skin. As soon as the opening of the needle has disappeared, the plunger is pushed down to drive in a little of the solution. A white swelling instantly forms in the tissues, which take on the aspect of "orange skin." One or more wheals, according to requirements, are thus marked out, and through them the needles are subsequently introduced for all the necessary injections.

Each injection should be made into the skin proper, without passage through into the subcutaneous cellular tissue, which is made evident by disappearance of resistance to the needle. If the skin of the region is delicate and movable, a fold of it should be taken up between the left thumb and index finger and the needle introduced at the top of this fold, meanwhile firmly held. The pain is very slight and evanescent, disappearing as soon as the anesthetic solution has been injected.

Injection at Right Angles.—When it is necessary to make an incision at right angles, as for blood transfusion, the intradermal injections of Reclus are superfluous, subcutaneous injection being sufficient to anesthetize the subcutaneous tissue. An intradermal wheal is made at one end of the incision; then, with a syringe provided with a long needle, an injection is made through the wheal, *under the skin,* the needle being inserted parallel to the surface in the subcutaneous tissues to the full length of the proposed incision or the distance that the needle permits. Inadvertent emergence of the point of the needle from within

outward should be avoided, as it is more painful
· than entrance of the needle from without in.

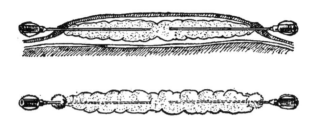

Fig. 7.—Subcutaneous infiltration of a straight band of skin
through two dermal wheals at either extremity. (*Reclus.*) A
needle traverses the dermal wheals without pain when the injection is made slowly. One mil of procaine-adrenin solution to
each centimeter of distance. The illustration presents both a
front and a side view, with curved or angular incisions.

After a few minutes the skin covering the injected tissue will have become insensible, the solution having anesthetized not only the subcutaneous

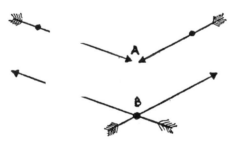

Fig. 8.—(*A*) The injections can be made through 2 wheals
or 1 wheal. (*B*) Continuous line of injections, as indicated
by the directions of the arrows. (*Pauchet.*)

tissue, but also the nerve filaments of the adjacent
skin. This is the simplest form of local anesthesia.

If one injection or one needle-length is not
sufficient, one should make two wheals, one at

each extremity of the proposed incision—or as many as may be required—and infiltrate from the·

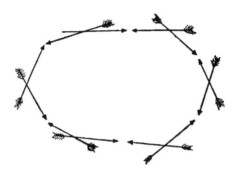

Fig. 9.—Injections surrounding a field of operation. (*Reclus.*) The 6 wheals are united by bands of infiltration as indicated by the arrows.

two ends (Fig. 7). Curved incisions or injections at right angles require an injection at the summit of the curve or angle, or two injections (Fig. 8).

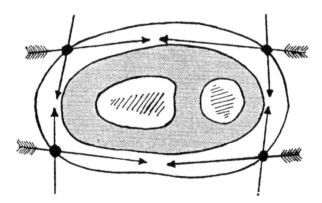

Fig. 10.—Shows the method of infiltrating the curved surface of the forearm through 4 dermal wheals, each wheal being placed at the summit of the curve. (*Pauchet.*) The injections are made in the directions shown by the arrows.

The curvature of the body surface prevents the penetration of a needle at right angles into the skin at a single injection. Thus, in injecting the subcutaneous tissues around the forearm, four wheals through each of which the needles are entered from both sides (Figs. 9 and 10) are required.

Infiltration of a subcutaneous band perpendicular to the axis of the limb anesthetizes not only the skin immediately covering the injected tissue,

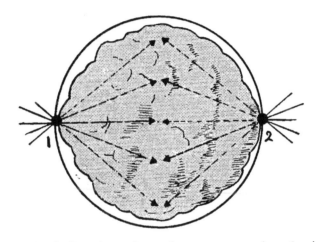

Fig. 11.—Infiltration of a subcutaneous surface by injections radiating from dermal wheals 1 and 2 (for the removal of skin grafts, excision of a chancroid, etc.). (*Pauchet.*)

but also all the subcutaneous tissues situated distally to the injected region (*circular anesthesia*).

Surface Infiltration.—This consists in the infiltration of an area of subcutaneous tissue by 1, 2, or more wheals. Through each of these points a long needle is introduced in all directions, anesthetizing the whole of the cutaneous surface bounded by the wheals. This procedure is serviceable for the preparation of Thiersch skin grafts (Fig. 11).

For the removal of skin tumors, subcutaneous infiltration of the base of the neoplasm suffices, without injection of the tumor itself (Fig. 12).

Anesthesia of Mucous Membranes.—The same directions hold good in the case of mucous membranes, but the wheals are unnecessary. One simply makes a sub-membranous injection, which renders the adjacent area of mucous membrane insensible.

Circular Injections.—In certain parts of the body the sensory nerves of the skin and of the

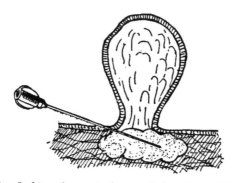

Fig. 12.—Infiltration of the pedicle of a skin tumor (molluscum). (*Pauchet.*)

fascia are continuous. Large portions of the body surface do not have special nerves from the sub-aponeurotic region. Hence it is not always necessary, in anesthetizing the skin and subcutaneous tissues, to inject the cellular tissue; in many instances a subcutaneous injection *surrounding* the latter suffices. This is what is termed *circular injection* (Fig. 13). At 1 and 2, two injections are made; the subcutaneous tissue is infiltrated from 1 to 3, 1 to 4, 2 to 3, and finally from 2 to 4, so that the operative field is surrounded by a subcutaneous wall of infiltration in the form of an elongated lozenge. The long diameter of the lozenge-shaped area corresponds to the direction of the incision to be subsequently made. Injections may instead be made at 3 and 4, if it is more

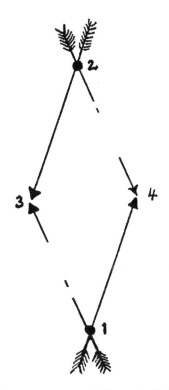

Fig. 13.—Subcutaneous quadrilateral infiltration through 1 and 2, in the shape of a lozenge, 1, 2, 3, and 4, following the direction of the arrows. (*Reclus.*)

convenient. The wall surrounding the operative field may, as desired, be made in the shape of a square, circle, etc. The number of wheals to be prepared for the injections depends upon the shape and dimensions of the operative field (Fig. 9).

In some parts of the body, the sensory nerves

run a prolonged subcutaneous course, supplying both the surface and the deep tissues. As regards the upper part of the head, the sensory nerves of the skin, pericranium, periosteum, and bones *all* course through the subcutaneous tissue at the level of the base of the cranium and forehead.

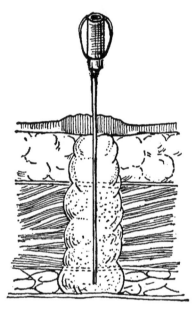

Fig. 14.—Anesthesia for tapping, as in ascites or pleurisy, or for the introduction of a radium tube into a tumor. (*Reclus.*)

Consequently a simple circular subcutaneous injection will desensitize large areas on the head, including the bones. Anesthesia of a finger is instituted on the same principle. The subcutaneous tissue of the first phalanx contains all the nerves of the finger. If a ring be injected around the base of the finger, the entire finger will be desensitized.

Deep Infiltration.—Simple circular subcutaneous injections are adequate only in parts of the body in which the nerve supply is disposed as in the parts above mentioned. They are *not* adequate when the nerve supply is deeply seated. Thus, on the chin, circular injection of an operative field in the center of which emerges the mental nerve would yield only an incomplete anesthesia. One of the primary essentials in inducing regional anesthesia is a systematic infiltration of any thick bed of tissue composed of different layers. An example of such anesthesia in its simplest form is that of the line of puncture in ascites or pleural effusion (Fig. 14).

The point of the injection is marked by a wheal, a needle of a convenient length inserted, and an injection made without interruption down to the subpleural or subperitoneal tissues. The pleural and the peritoneal nerves require separate infiltration because they course in the subpleural or subperitoneal tissues.

Infiltration by Layers.—A systematic infiltration of a mass of tissues is that which will act upon all the layers of tissue therein contained (Fig. 15). One should begin with deep injections and finish with subcutaneous ones. The needle, through a wheal, is inserted in a perpendicular direction to the deepest point. It is then brought up to the subcutaneous tissue and inserted again, injecting *obliquely* toward the middle of the tissue-mass to be infiltrated, and so on. The last injection is made in a parallel direction under the skin. The fluid is injected continuously during the introduction and withdrawal of the needle. If the length of the needle will allow, a single wheal at one extremity or in the middle suffices.

At no point in the body are subperiosteal injections necessary for desensitization of the periosteum, which receives its nerves from without and becomes desensitized through the influence of the fluid in the tissues which cover it.

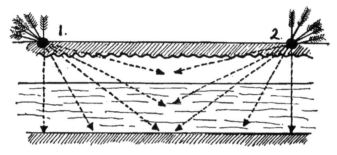

Fig. 15.—Osteotomy of the femur. (*Pauchet.*) Anesthesia of the diaphysis. Make two wheals, 1 and 2. From these two points make the injections above and below as shown by the arrows, forming a liquid sheath round the periosteum. If the ears of the patient be stopped with cotton, one may saw or break the bone without causing him pain or nervous disturbance.

Infiltration of thick masses of tissues, as just described, demands a certain amount of practice. One must learn to feel with the point of the needle. One must know at every instant which anatomical layer is being entered. The hand soon becomes accustomed to recognizing when the needle-point is traversing a resistant layer and when it again passes into a layer of soft tissues. Injection through the muscular aponeuroses generally causes slight pain. Therefore, one should inject the fluid progressively as the needle is being introduced, following the method of Reclus. By this procedure injection of a large amount of the anesthetic into a vein is obviated, while at the same time, continuous injection insures an equal distribution of the solution. When an injection

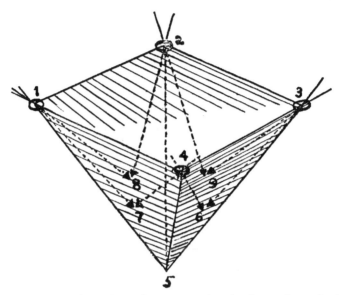

Fig. 16.—Infiltration of a layer of soft tissue through dermal wheals 1 and 2. (*Pauchet.*) The injections follow the direction of the arrows down to the bone, the last made being those entering the subcutaneous cellular tissue.

in the proximity of large vessels is required, it is best to introduce the needle independently of the syringe and to inject the fluid only if blood fails to flow from the needle lumen. Puncture of a large artery or vein, is, of course, to be avoided, but it is altogether free of danger if fine needles are employed.

Injection of a small area suffices whenever a simple incision in healthy tissue is alone required, *e.g.,* for the extraction of a foreign body from a definitely known situation.

Regional anesthesia likewise permits of securing insensibility of large fields of operation.

Often infiltration of a single locality will destroy sensation in most of the nerves leading to the field of operation. This is the case, *e.g.,* in operations at the front of the neck, or for the cure of femoral or inguinal hernia. At other

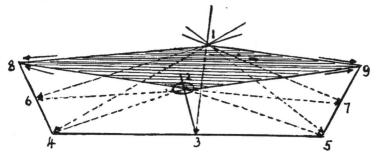

Fig. 17.—Pyramidal injections. (*Pauchet.*) Through the dermal wheals 1, 2, 3, and 4, one may painlessly infiltrate four triangular layers, union of which isolates a pyramid of anesthetized tissue. (Removal of a shell fragment, etc.)

times, one must infiltrate simultaneously all the layers surrounding the operative field.

The technique will be readily understood upon inspection of a few diagrams.

Fig. 16 represents a pyramid. Its summit, 5, is deeply situated beneath the center of the operative field, while its base, 1, 2, 3, and 4, is at the cutaneous surface. Its lateral surfaces bound the field of operation; it is these sides which require to be injected.

Dermal wheals, 1, 2, 3, and 4, are first marked out. Through each of these a long needle is introduced at first toward point 5, then toward various points situated on the lateral surfaces, *e.g.,* from 1 to 7, 4 to 7, 4 to 6, 3 to 6, 3 to 9, 2 to 9, etc. The field of operation thus becomes desensitized without having been directly reached by

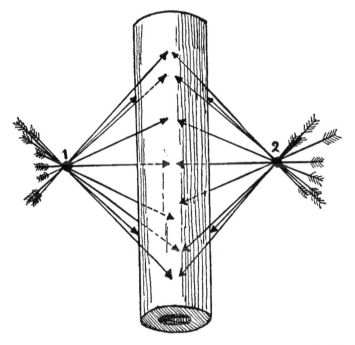

Fig. 18.—Boat-shaped infiltration through dermal wheals 1 and 2. Injection of four quadrilateral surfaces, permitting the removal of a tumor or foreign body. (*Pauchet.*)

the anesthetic. Often two surface injections suffice to encompass the area perfectly. In other cases. more than four are required, and the designs for injection assume, according to the extent of the operative field, many varied forms: cone, base of a cone, a boat-shaped solid, etc. In Fig. 17 there are two points of entrance, viz.,

1 and 2, through which one injects toward 3, 4, 5, 6, and 7, and finally infiltrates the subcutaneous tissue. Fig. 18 shows a field of operation on a limb; by the type of anesthesia depicted the bone may be desensitized. For all these injections a ½ per cent. solution is used. A more concentrated solution, from 1 per cent. to 4 per cent., injected in small amounts, is preferable wherever large quantities of liquid would lead to difficulty or discomfort, as in the orbit, eyelids, foreskin (circumcision), fingers, etc.

Small amounts of these concentrated solutions oftentimes exert a prolonged effect. Injection of a small quantity of anesthetic may affect not only the region injected but also the trunk of a nerve supplying surfaces at a distance.

Perineural or Endoneural Injection by the Subcutaneous Route.—Anesthesia of a large nerve-trunk is often combined with peripheral infiltration, and is governed by certain definite principles. In the first place, the point of the needle must be brought in contact with the nerve. This is readily done whenever the nerve is situated near a bone constituting a landmark, as in the case of the ulnar nerve, but is more difficult when such landmarks are absent and when the nerve is situated in the midst of soft tissues. One of the most reliable indications of the needle reaching the nerve is afforded by a paresthesia radiating toward the periphery. The sharp pain referred in the direction of the nerve distribution demonstrates the contact of the needle with the nerve.

The patient should therefore be told of this before the needle is introduced and should let the operator know as soon as the paresthesia is experienced.

For the injection of large nerves it is well to use from 1 to 5 mils of a concentrated solution, 2 to 4 per cent., of procaine-adrenin.

The length of time one must wait after having made the injection depends upon the manner in which the nerve has been reached. If the needle has been introduced into the nerve root, as occurs in the case of the fifth nerve, abolition of sensation is instantaneous. If the anesthetic has merely been injected around the nerve trunk, 5 to 20 minutes elapse before complete insensibility is established.

Direct Endoneural Injection.—Exposed nerve-trunks may be desensitized by the injection of a little 4 per cent. solution—viz., 1 ampoule—using a 3-centimeter needle. This procedure is very satisfactory for operations on nerves. The operator begins by incising the layers of tissues covering the nerve, as these have already been injected with procaine-adrenin. When the nerve has been located beneath the incision, he injects directly into the trunk the contents of a 2-mil ampoule of the 4 per cent. solution.

Choice of Procedure.—The nature of the affection to be operated for—wound, removal of foreign body or of an inflammatory or neoplastic tumor—governs the form of the injection, and one must always be careful to desensitize a large enough area in order to be prepared for all eventualities and have a certain degree of latitude during the operation. One should avoid injecting the line of incision, and keep always at a certain distance from diseased tissues, particularly if infected. A well defined furuncle should be encircled by an injection in the form of a pyramid, at quite a distance from the inflamed tissues. Diffuse phlegmons lend themselves to local anesthesia only if it is possible to desensitize them at a distance from the field of operation. Malignancy of a tumor is no contraindication to regional anesthesia if the entire field can be desensitized without an injection in contact with the tumor. One must not forget the temporary ischemia which adrenin produces in the infiltrated area. This ischemia is often an advantage, as it reduces hemorrhage to the point of totally changing the aspect of certain operations, such as those for hemorrhoids, resection of the superior maxillary or of the tongue, laryngectomy, etc. But in plastic operations one must be careful not to ischemize the base of the flap to be turned back, as this would compromise its vitality.

For plastic operations of the face, strong solutions of procaine without adrenin should be used; the solution runs out with the blood, and the anesthesia need not last long, as these operations are always of short duration.

CHAPTER III.

CRANIAL OPERATIONS.

THE sensory nerves supplying the skin of the forehead, the temples, and the scalp, all pass at the level of a line encircling the skull from the eyelids to the external occipital protuberance (Fig. 19). From there they branch ‑to the summit of

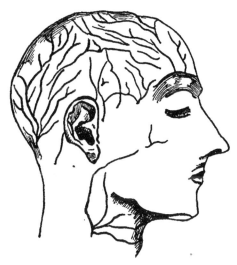

Fig. 19.—Nerve supply of the scalp. (*Hirschfeld.*) Injection of a 1 per cent. solution of procaine-adrenin on a line completely surrounding the head above the ears and eyebrows completely desensitizes the nerve supply to the scalp.

the cranium, where they spread out under the skin and the cranial aponeurosis. It is therefore very easy to anesthetize the entire cranium by a circular injection at this line. The nerves referred to supply not only the skin and pericranium, but also the bones of the summit of the cranium and their periosteum. The dura mater is not sensitive to pain except below the base of the skull; therefore operations upon the summit are painless.

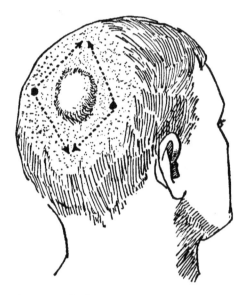

Fig. 20.—Tumor of the scalp. (*Pauchet.*) Whether the condition be a wen, a lipoma, or a sarcoma of the cranium, infiltration of the epicranium induces complete anesthesia. The illustration shows a lozenge-shaped injection circumscribing the tumor through dermal wheals in accordance with the direction of the arrows.

A simple circular injection under the skin suffices for trephining and operations on the brain.

Where muscles, however, cover the cranial bones at the line of injection, they must be injected. A band of infiltration, starting in front from the eyelids, extending to the occiput, and passing above the arch of the ear, will desensitize the entire cranium above this line. It is not necessary to make a subperiosteal injection. The band of anesthesia just mentioned possesses another advantage: The cranial arteries ascend, like the nerves, spreading out toward the summit under the epicranium or, as in the case of the

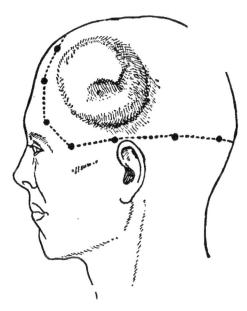

Fig. 21.—Craniectomy for sarcoma. (*Braun.*) The frontal portion of the infiltration is designed to abolish sensibility of the anastomoses between the frontal and parietal nerves.

temporal arteries, in the muscles. Adrenin contracts them, rendering the operative field relatively bloodless, and the various methods for arresting hemorrhage superfluous. At times the large arteries bleed a little and must be clamped; the small arteries do not bleed. For small fields of operation a ½ per cent. solution suffices; for large fields, rich in vessels, a 1 per cent. will yield a better hemostasis.

Starting from two wheals which correspond, respectively, to the extremities of the intended incision, one injects in a lozenge or quadrilateral form 10 to 20 mils of a ½ per cent. solution (Figs. 20, 21, 22).

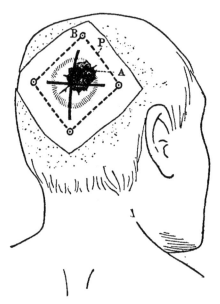

Fig. 22.—Anesthesia for trephining. (*Pauchet.*) Observe the crucial incision. *A*, the wound. *B*, dermal wheals. *P*, a zone of infiltration 1 centimeter in width surrounding the wound, as shown by the dotted line down to the bone. This yields perfect anesthesia and ischemia.

Treatment of Large Wounds in the Soft Tissues, or of Compound Fractures, of the Skull.

Several wheals are made around the wound—as in Fig. 23, in which there are seven—sufficiently close together for the curvature of the skull to permit of the needle going under the epicranium. With a 1 per cent. solution, a narrow band of infiltration, circumscribing the field of operation according to the line indicated, is now traced in the soft, subaponeurotic tissues. Along a distance of 5 centimeters, about 5 mils of solution should be injected.

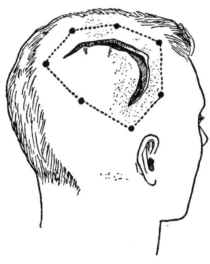

Fig. 23.—Anesthesia of the epicranium around a wound (*Pauchet.*) This can be practised in all operations upon the cranium for war wounds (bone and soft tissues) through as many dermal wheals as may be necessary to surround completely the territory with a zone of infiltration, made with a 1 per cent. solution.

The peripheral line of injection should be far enough removed from the wound to permit of all necessary excision or enlargement for perfect repair, for any pedicle required or for a dissection necessary for plastic repair. Only a few moments are required for complete anesthesia.

In their ambulance on the western fighting front, in September, 1914, Pauchet and Labouré trephined a case for hemiplegia, under local anesthesia, with the patient in the sitting position. After the completion of the operation the patient walked to the railway station, assisted by a fellow-soldier.

REMOVAL OF MALIGNANT TUMORS OF THE CRANIUM, WITH BONE RESECTION.

The surgeon required to remove a tumor adherent to the skull should at the same time remove the skin covering the tumor and a rather

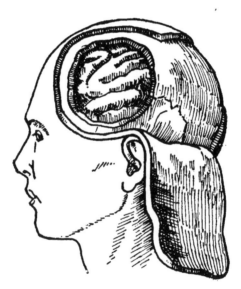

Fig. 24.—Repair of a craniectomy. (*Braun.*) Shows a flap to be re-applied as covering to the bony surface excised. It is well to cover the opening over the brain with a layer of fascia lata to replace the dura mater and prevent adhesions of the skin to the deeper surfaces. Skin grafts may be used to cover the denuded occipital zone when new tissue has grown over the skull. The opening in the skull should be reinforced with a chondrocostal piece or a gold plate. All this may be perfectly done under local anesthesia.

large section of bone. The operation will be painless, since the dura mater, together with all the other local tissues, are insensitive. The anesthesia should be instituted as already indicated, viz., on a line extending from the eyes to the occipital protuberance, the line of the hat band.

Equally good results are obtained in the case of a sarcoma originating in the periosteum and adhering to the skin. The surgeon is enabled to remove painlessly the skin, pericranium, periosteum, bone tissues, and dura mater. The brain surface should under these conditions be recovered with skin. The liberation of an area of skin posteriorly for this purpose may likewise be effected without pain.

Trephining the Temporal Region.

Regional anesthesia permits of removal of epidural hematomas of the inferior meninges, craniectomy for decompression (Babinski), and removal of bone fragments and foreign bodies. The dura mater near the base of the cranium is sensitive, but only moderately so.

Fig. 25 shows how to place the wheals, and the form of the injection, for the dissection of a temporal osteocutaneous flap.

One is in the middle of the superior border of the zygoma; at this point one injects subcutaneously a ½ or 1 per cent. solution. There is also to be infiltrated a layer of temporal muscle as shown in the diagrammatic Fig. 26, represent-

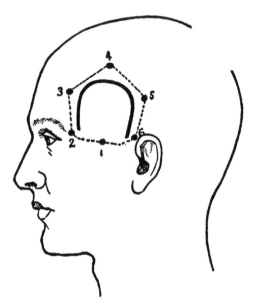

Fig. 25.—Trephining the temporal region for decompression, (*Pauchet.*) The horse-shoe-shaped flap comprises the skin, the temporal muscle, and the periosteum. The illustration shows the surrounding band of anesthesia induced through six dermal wheals. The lower side of the pentagon, wheals 1, 2, and 6, should be infiltrated down to the bone with a 1 per cent. solution of procaine-adrenin; the other sides, with a ½ per cent. solution.

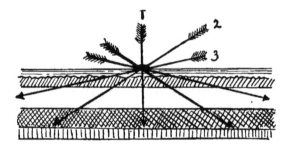

Fig. 26.—Anesthesia of the base of the pentagon (Fig. 25) for trephining the temporal region. (*Pauchet.*) The fan-shaped infiltration follows the direction of the arrows. Arrows 1 and 2 pierce the temporal muscle and reach the bone; arrow 3 infiltrates the subcutaneous tissue.

ing a horizontal incision parallel to the superior
border of the zygoma through the skin, temporal

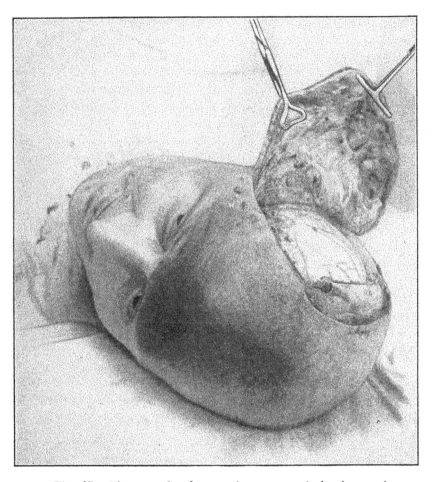

Fig. 27.—Photograph of a craniectomy made in the service
of Dr. Babinski. (*Pauchet.*) The musculo-cutaneous flap is
held by two clamps; note that the operation is practically
bloodless on account of the adrenin contained in the solution
injected. The dura mater is not opened.

muscle and temporal bone. The needle is first
introduced through wheal 1, perpendicularly
from the surface down to the bone (arrow 1)

then obliquely toward the anterior and posterior
margins of the temporal muscle, again down to
the bone (arrow 2) and following a horizontal
plane, and finally even more obliquely in the subcutaneous tissue (arrow 3), from 2 to 6. To infiltrate this layer, about 30 mils is required; to
circumscribe the field of operation, about 30 mils
more; in all, about 60 mils of procaine-adrenin
solution.

Removal of the Gasserian ganglion would be
practicable by this method, but at the present time
injection of the branches of the 5th nerve at their
emergence from the ganglion, and their destruc-
tion by alcohol, is preferred.

Exposure of the Cerebellum.

In 1912 we suggested to Thierry de Martel
the following technique, which this skillful operator was the first to apply in tumor of the cerebellum with complete success. Fig. 28 shows the
situation of the wheals and the shape of the incision for exposing the cerebellar hemispheres. It
is best not to depart from this tracing, even if
one has decided not to touch more than half of
the cerebellum. Points 3 and 9 are placed just
behind the base of the mastoid. From these two
points, as from 1, 2, and 10, the necessary injections are made in the muscles of the neck. Next,
the muscular layer outlined by the points of injection is impregnated with a solution of procaine-
adrenin along the line shown. In the flap itself

no injection is made. This illustration, taken in conjunction with that for temporal injection (Fig. 26), defines the path of the needle. The point should penetrate to the transverse processes of the cervical vertebræ and down to the occiput. Union of the successive injections by subcutaneous injec-

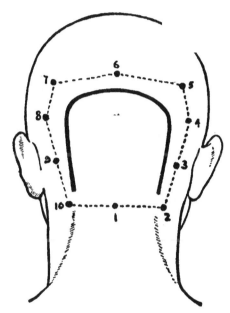

Fig. 28.—Trephining for a tumor of the cerebellum. (*Pauchet.*) The 10 dermal wheals in the form of a trapezium surround the field of operation with a zone of infiltration. The proposed flap is shown by the dark line in the shape of a horse-shoe.

tions follows; 100 to 120 mils of solution are used, over half of which goes into the muscles of the neck. Thierry de Martel operated with his patient sitting astride a chair, with the arms resting on its back, and his head resting on his arms. The dura mater of the posterior cerebral fossæ and the cerebellum are insensitive to pain.

CHAPTER IV.

ANESTHESIA OF THE HEAD AND NECK.

THE surgery of the head and the neck is of interest both to general operators and, particularly, to three classes of specialists, the ophthalmologist, the otorhinolaryngologist, and the stomatologist.

In these regions the sensory supply is furnished by the fifth nerve and the cervical plexus. The fifth nerve is predominant in the face. As several branches often combine in supplying sensation to a single region, it is sometimes necessary in these tissues to combine root or trunk anesthesia with peripheral infiltration. Or, it may be necessary to combine root anesthesia with anesthesia of the neighboring regions.

We shall first consider synthetically the subject of anesthesia of the nerve roots and nerve branches, and then describe the technique for each operation involved in the three specialties mentioned.

ANESTHESIA OF THE GASSERIAN GANGLION.

The ganglion of the fifth nerve is intracranial. It rests upon the summit of the petrous portion' of the temporal bone (Fig. 29) in a fold of the dura mater just above and behind the foramen ovale, and in the immediate neighborhood of a

(48)

venous sinus and of the motor nerves of the eye (fourth and sixth). It has three branches: the ophthalmic, the superior maxillary, and the inferior maxillary. The ganglion is accessible through the foramen ovale, an orifice measuring ½ centimeter by 2 or 3 millimeters. This foramen is situated on the floor of the cranium immediately

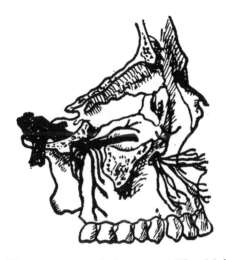

Fig. 29.—The ganglion of Gasser. (*Hirschfeld.*) It rests upon the summit of the petrous portion of the temporal bone. From above downward the illustration shows the origin of the ophthalmic nerve and of the superior and inferior maxillary nerves.

behind the base of the pterygoid process. It corresponds, for the superior maxillary, to the outer side of the last two molars in the sagittal region. It is located at a depth of 45 millimeters from the zygoma.

Indications for Gasserian anesthesia are two in number:

A. Surgical operations on the face.

4

B. Alcoholization of the nerve to combat persistent neuralgia (Sicard).

The anesthetist should bear in mind the following precepts:

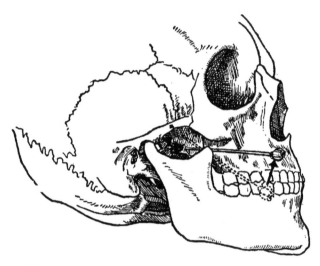

Fig. 30.—Injection of the Gasserian ganglion through the foramen ovale. (*Braun.*) (1) The needle represented by the dotted lines is introduced 3 centimeters from the commissure of the lips, in the direction of the zygomatic arch, until it reaches the subtemporal region between the two maxillary bones. (2) The black line needle shows the shank raised and the needle directed toward the zygomatic tubercle. Being kept in contact with the bone, it reaches the foramen ovale, coming in contact with the fifth nerve, in the terminal branches of which it provokes pain.

(1) Use a fine, sharp, flexible, but strong needle.

(2) Inject slowly.

(3) Employ a concentrated solution in small quantities, viz., 1 to 2 mils of a 2 or 4 per cent. solution of procaine-adrenin.

In spite of these precautions, vertigo, vomiting and even symptoms of meningitis are sometimes observed.   These post-anesthetic disturbances do

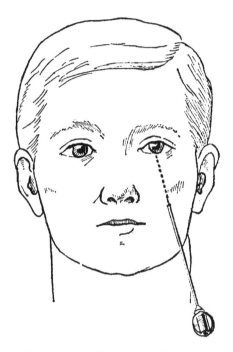

Fig. 31.—Injection of the Gasserian ganglion (*Braun.*) The patient should sit erect, looking directly forward.   The surgeon introduces the needle through the cheek 3 centimeters from the labial commissure, so directing it that it remains in the plane of the subject's pupil.   The index finger of the left hand is introduced into the patient's mouth to make certain that the needle shall not pierce the mucous membrane.   The needle should be directed between the inferior maxillary and the tuberosity of the superior maxillary.

not detract from the value of the procedure because the method of anesthesia under discussion is employed for serious operations on the face, or obstinate neuralgia of the fifth nerve, which warrant its application.

Technique of the Injection.—The patient may be in the lying or sitting position. Injection is easier on a sitting subject, the operator standing or sitting in front of the patient. A needle 9 centimeters in length should be selected.

The landmarks include some that are appre-

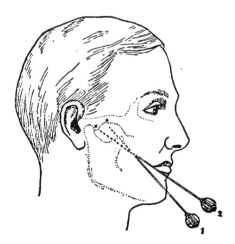

Fig. 32.—Injection of the Gasserian ganglion. (*Braun*). The same maneuver as in the preceding illustration. The needle is first directed at the middle of the zygomatic arch. As soon as the point touches the bone of the subtemporal region, the shank is raised so that the point is directed at the zygomatic tubercle. Being then pushed forward about 1 centimeter, it will penetrate the foramen ovale.

ciable to sight or palpation and others which are found by the point of the needle as it is introduced.

(1) When the subject looks straight to the front the pupil of the eye supplies the direction of the frontal plane in which the needle must be directed.   •

(2) The labial fissure.

(3) The second upper molar.

(4) The ascending ramus of the inferior maxillary, the inner surface of which may be felt by introducing the index finger into the mouth.

(5) The tuberosity of the superior maxillary.

(6) The bone in the subtemporal region; the needle, when correctly directed, will strike against

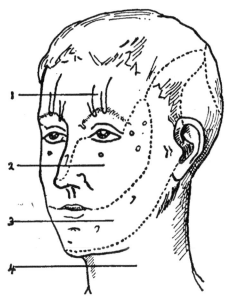

Fig. 33.—The sensory nerve supply of the face and neck. (*Hirschfeld.*) (1) Ophthalmic. (2) Superior maxillary. (3) Inferior maxillary. (4) Cervical plexus (anterior branches).

this resistant surface, which is situated in front of the foramen ovale.

(7) The middle of the zygomatic arch and the tubercle of the zygoma; the tubercle indicates the point at which the needle must be directed in order to enter the foramen; the middle of the arch indicates the bony region anterior to the foramen against which the needle must strike before penetrating the foramen (Figs. 30, 31, 32).

The cheek is pierced 3 centimeters beyond the labial fissure, on a line with the lobe of the ear. The needle is inserted with one hand. With the index finger of the other in the mouth, the second

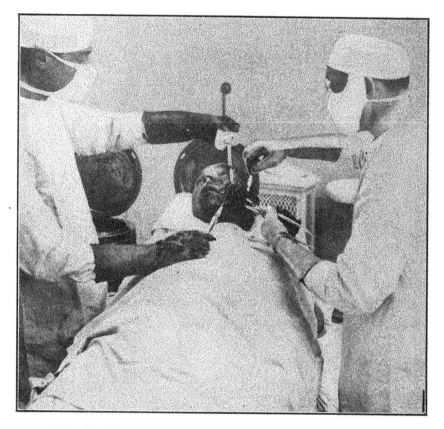

Fig. 34.—Removal of a cancer from the velum palati and left tonsil by transverse incision of the cheek and resection of the ascending ramus of the inferior maxillary bone after anesthesia of the Gasserian ganglion. (*Pauchet.*) The photograph shows the loosening of the upper fragment of the inferior maxillary, operated upon by *Pauchet* and *Sourdat.*

superior molar and the tuberosity of the superior maxillary are located within, and the ascending ramus of the mandible without. The needle is to pass in the interval bounded by these .bones; the finger in the mouth follows the needle point under the mucous membrane and prevents it from perforating the latter.

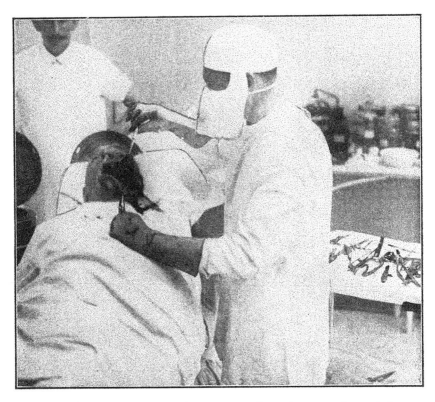

Fig. 35.—The wound is held open after the resection of the maxillary has been completed. (*Pauchet.*)

One next aims at the subtemporal region to strike the bony surface already mentioned. The needle should be directed somewhat obliquely inward, *i.e.,* in the line of the pupil when the subject is looking straight ahead. It should be also slightly oblique upward, *i.e.,* should virtually pass through the middle of the zygoma,—which can be

controlled by surveying the patient in profile. Its
point should be behind the second upper molar.
Thus directed, the needle enters the subtemporal
region, which marks the end of the first stage of

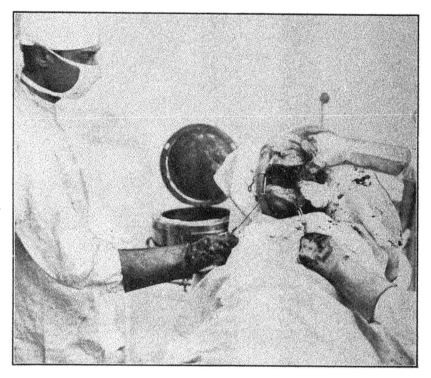

Fig. 36.—The tonsillar space is tamponed after the resection of a part of the pharynx and of the tongue. The borders
of the incised cheek are retracted, showing the extent of the
wound. The tongue is drawn out with the aid of a cord held
by the assistant.

the injection. Care should be taken to do all this
very slowly, in order not to blunt the point of
the needle by contact with the bone.

Then the point is disengaged and, slightly
raising the shank but still remaining in the plane
of the pupil, the point is advanced about 1 centi-

meter, gliding along the surface of the subtemporal bone. In profile one aims this time for the tubercle of the zygoma. Resistance ceases as the needle enters the foramen ovale. A tense membrane is traversed about 7 centimeters beneath the skin. When the patient notices radiating pains at first in the superior maxillary nerve, entrance into the ganglion is indicated. One should then inject 1 to 1½ mils of a 2 per cent. procaine-adrenin, very slowly and gently pushing the needle in another ½ centimeter.

By the same route, but without entering the foramen ovale, one may reach the inferior maxillary nerve as it emerges from this foramen and limit the injection to it. It is difficult clearly to describe this procedure in words, and we have therefore attempted to supplement the explanation and more fully guide the operator by the several appended cuts.

ANESTHESIA OF THE OPHTHALMIC NERVE.

The frontal, internal and external nasal, and lachrymal nerves separate from the origin of the ophthalmic immediately before it enters the orbit. The ophthalmic is fan-shaped and is situated between the bony plate and the muscular cone of the orbit; the injection must, therefore, be made between these two. The frontal and lachrymal nerves are situated externally and emerge through the superior orbital fissure. They are reached along the external wall of the orbit.

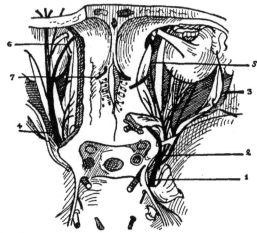

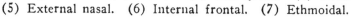

Fig. 37.—The ophthalmic nerve and its branches. (*Testut.*)
(1) Ophthalmic. (2) Nasal. (3) Lachrymal. (4) Frontal.
(5) External nasal. (6) Internal frontal. (7) Ethmoidal.

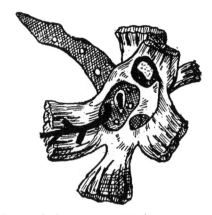

Fig. 38.—Base of the orbit. (*Testut.*) Zinn's ring, where
the motor muscles of the eye are attached. On the left is
seen the sphenoidal fissure in the center of Zinn's ring. The
nasal nerve and ophthalmic vein are in the ring. The frontal,
lachrymal, and pathetic nerves are in the sphenoidal fissure.

The nasal nerves occupy the upper internal angle of the orbit, and are infiltrated at that point.

The frontal nerves supply sensation to a triangular area of integument with its base corresponding to the entire frontal region above the

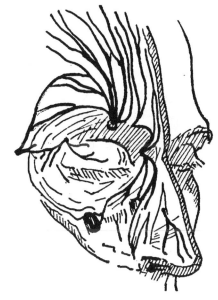

Fig. 39.—Supraorbital branches of the ophthalmic nerve. (*Hirschfeld.*) To anesthetize these branches, inject parallel to the superior border of the orbit.

root of the nose and its apex at the scalp (Fig. 40). They also sensitize the frontal sinuses and the upper eyelids. The nasal nerves supply the frontal, ethmoidal, and sphenoidal sinuses, the nasal septum, and the nasal lobes.

Injections may be made from three points, according to the operation required.

(*a*) *Frontal Infiltration.*—The operator injects under the skin 10 mils of a 1 per cent. procaine-adrenin, commencing above the external orbital apophysis and ending above the corresponding apophysis on the opposite side. The line of injection is shown by the black line in Fig. 40.

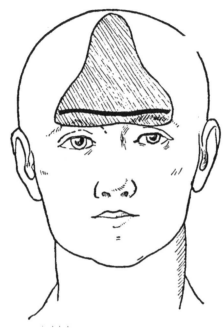

Fig. 40.—Injections along the black line anesthetize the ophthalmic branches of the fifth nerve and render insensible a triangular area. (*Pauchet* and *Sourdat.*)

(*b*) *External Orbital Infiltration.*—This blocks the frontal and lachrymal nerves.

The needle is introduced at the external angle and the outer wall of the orbit followed with its point. At a depth of about 4½ centimeters the needle point will come in contact with bone, the

orbital vault, and will have passed into the external portion of the sphenoidal fissure, where are situated the frontal and lachrymal nerves. Five mils
of the 2 per cent. solution are now injected, and
the resulting anesthesia will be complete (Figs.
41, 42).

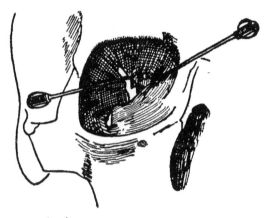

Fig. 41.—Intraorbital injections for infiltration of the
ophthalmic branches. (*Braun.*) To the left, an external injection, which keeps in contact with the external orbital wall.
At a depth of 4 centimeters the needle point strikes the orbital
vault. It now crosses the extremity of the sphenoidal fissure,
along which pass the lachrymal and nasal nerves. A 1 per
cent. solution of procaine-adrenin is injected.

To the right, an internal injection. The needle follows
the superointernal angle of the orbit, constantly in contact with
the bone and grazing the ethmoidal foramen. At a depth of 4
centimeters it comes in contact with the orbital vault. The
solution is injected while the needle is being introduced.

(*c*) *Internal Orbital Infiltration.*—At an equal
distance from the eyebrow and the caruncle, *i.e.,*
1 centimeter above the internal commissure of the
eyelids, the needle is introduced against the superior internal angle of the bony wall, which should

be continuously followed. At a depth of 4 or at
most 4½ centimeters, 5 mils of a 2 per cent. solution are injected (Figs. 41, 42).

This last injection anesthetizes the nasal wall
and the ethmoidal, sphenoidal, and frontal sinuses,
as well as the lobe of the nose. It induces

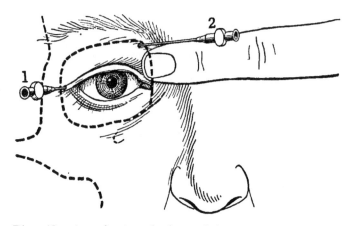

Fig. 42.—Anesthesia of the ophthalmic branches by the
orbital route: (1) External. (2) Internal. (*Pauchet.*) The
dotted line shows the shape and extent of the orbital orifice.
Needle 1 is entered at the extreme angle of the commissure of the eyelids. It follows the bony wall and stops only
when it comes in contact with the orbital vault, where it crosses
the sphenoidal fissure (see Fig. 41). Needle 2 is entered at
the superior internal border of the orbit, one finger breadth
above the caruncle. The point is kept in constant contact with
the superior internal angle of the bony wall to reach the
ethmoid nerves.

edema of the upper lid, causes projection of the
eye-ball, and sometimes results in blindness for a
few minutes. The optic nerve is not anesthetized.

ANESTHESIA OF THE SUPERIOR MAXILLARY NERVE.

The superior maxillary passes through the foramen rotundum at the bottom of the pterygomaxillary fissure, precisely between the tuberosity

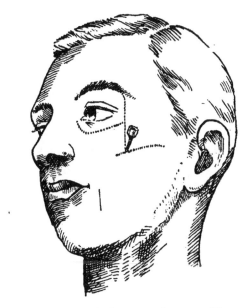

Fig. 43.—Injection of the superior maxillary at the foramen rotundum by the external route. (*Braun.*) The needle is introduced at the intersection of a vertical line drawn downward following the external border of the orbit and a line drawn along the inferior border of the superior maxillary bone (dotted lines).

of the superior maxillary and the base of the pterygoid process.

(*à*) *External Route* (Figs. 43, 44).—Locate the zygomatic arch with the finger; mark its lower border with ink; mark the external border of the orbit in the same manner at the point where a vertical line drawn from this external

border meets the zygomatic arch (just behind the
lower angle of the body of the malar bone), and
introduce the needle to a depth of 5 to 6 centimeters. In this way the nerve is reached at once;
but it is preferable to attain first, with the point
of the needle, the body of the maxillary on its
inclined surface, feeling one's way, and directing
the needle deeply. Suddenly the needle will come

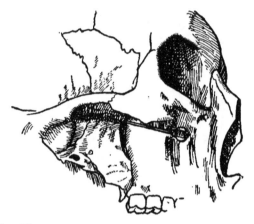

Fig. 44.—The needle is first directed toward the tuberosity
of the maxillary bone, whence it penetrates directly about 4
centimeters and enters the pterygo-maxillary fissure. (*Braun.*)
When the patient complains of a shooting pain in the teeth,
from 3 to 4 mils of a 2 per cent. anesthetic solution are injected.

to an empty space and touch the nerve, when the
patient will experience a sharp pain in the face
and upper teeth. Five mils of a 2 per cent. procaine-adrenin solution are now injected, and while
withdrawing the needle, 5 mils of a ½ per cent.
solution. To cause the branches of the internal
maxillary to contract, it is often necessary to have
the patient open his mouth, when the needle will
enter more easily (Fig. 45).

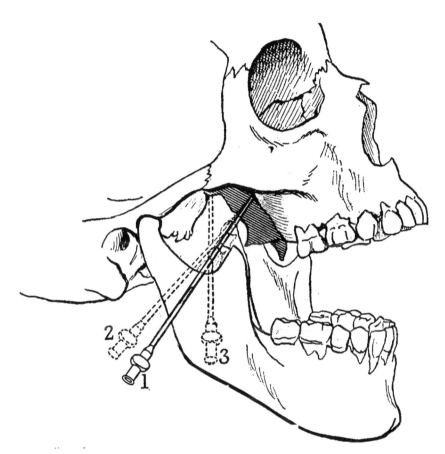

Fig. 45.—Anesthesia of the superior and inferior maxillary
through the same orifice. (*Pauchet.*) The patient is made to
open his mouth. The needle is introduced below the zygomatic arch and introduced as far as the pterygoid process, then
partly withdrawn and the point directed slightly forward to
reach the pterygo-maxillary fissure, where it encounters the
superior maxillary nerve at the foramen rotundum. Again the
needle is partly withdrawn and then reinserted about 1 centimeter further back, where it reaches the foramen ovale behind the root of the pterygoid process. The foramen ovale
is at a depth of about 4 to 5 centimeters.

(*b*) *Orbital Route* (Figs. 46, 47).—At· the junction of the external, lateral, and inferior borders of the orbit, a dermal wheal is made and the

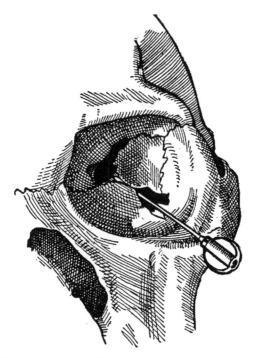

Fig. 46.—Anesthesia of the left superior maxillary nerve at the foramen rotundum by the orbital route. (*Braun.*) The needle, which at first is held vertically (Fig. 47), comes in contact with the floor of the orbit on a level with its inferior external angle. Entering deeper, it reaches a space on a level with the orbital ·fissure. Thence it progresses backward almost horizontally, following the direction of the fissure. At a ·depth of about 5 centimeters it reaches the base of the cranium and the foramen rotundum. One to 2 mils of a 2 per cent. anesthetic solution are injected.

point of the needle then introduced almost vertically downward. In order that it shall pass along the floor of the orbit, it should be directed

slightly backward.   At a depth of about 1 centimeter it will traverse a fibrous layer—the fissure
of the orbital floor.   As soon as the needle reaches
this space its flange end should be lowered so as
to bring it almost horizontal, while the head of

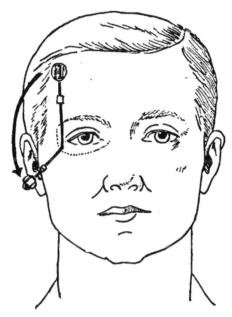

Fig. 47.—This figure shows the manner in which the needle
point is made to follow the floor of the orbit. By placing a
rubber shield upon the needle, the surgeon can make the latter serve as an index of depth in the procedure described in
Fig. 46.   (*Braun.*)

the patient is held quite erect.   If the needle is not
horizontal, it will enter the subtemporal space.
Yet it should not be introduced too high up, or
it will enter the eyeball.   It should be directed in
the plane of the fissure, *i.e.,* in the direction of
the inferior, external angle.   One should always

feel a certain resistance at this point. At a depth
of 5 centimeters, the situation of the needle will
correspond to the foramen rotundum. At this
point it will come in contact with the base of the
skull. Five mils of a 2 per cent. solution of neo-

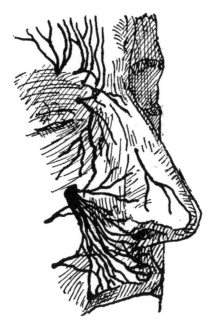

Fig. 48.—Emergence of the infraorbital nerve. (*Hirschfeld.*) On the same vertical line as the supraorbital nerve, it
is situated ½ centimeter below the middle of the lower border
of the orbital foramen.

caine-adrenin are now injected. At times a temporary paralysis of the muscles of the eye, or a
hematoma in the pterygomaxillary fissure, will appear. Both these conditions are incidents devoid
of serious consequences.

ANESTHESIA OF THE INFRAORBITAL NERVE.

The infraorbital nerve, a branch of the superior maxillary, is accessible through the cheek. The lower border of the orbit is marked with a dermal pencil, a line drawn from the center downward ½ centimeter, and a cross made. This corresponds to the point of emergence of the infraorbital nerve. The three apertures whence the infraorbital and mental nerves arise are on the same vertical line, and correspond to the interval between the first and second premolars (Fig. 45). A dermal wheal is made, and the subcutaneous cellular tissues infiltrated so that contact will not be painful. Then, with the needle, the infraorbital opening is found. Coming in contact with the bone, the operator feels around while directing the needle a little higher and outward; soon he becomes aware of a small depression and penetrates into a canal. The patient feels a sharp pain. One mil of a 2 per cent. solution is now injected. The anesthesia thus induced extends to the lower lid, the upper lip, the nasal ala, a part of the skin and mucous membrane of the cheek, the mucous membrane of the lips, the margins of the superior alveolar process, as well as the inferior walls of the superior maxillary and the incisor and canine teeth.

Anesthesia of the Superior Dental Nerves.

(a) *Buccal Route.*—The zygomatic arch is located through the mouth. When its most anterior point is felt, the mucous membrane is pierced and the needle introduced for a distance of 1 or 2 centimeters. The patient will usually feel pain in his teeth. Five mils of a 2 per cent. procaine-adrenin solution are now injected.

(b) *External Route.*—The zygomatic arch is located and the same route followed as that taken to reach the superior maxillary nerve. As soon as the tuberosity of the superior maxillary is attained, 5 mils of solution are injected. This injection anesthetizes the upper molars and premolars as well as the mucous membrane of the maxillary sinus (Fig. 29).

Anesthesia of the Nerves of the Palate.

The inferior palatine nerve emerges from the posterior palatine canal above the last molar. The nasopalatine nerve arises in the anterior palatine canal, in the median line and behind the incisors. The needle is introduced anteriorly, under the mucous membrane of the palate, immediately behind the teeth and in the median line. One mil of a 2 per cent. procaine-adrenin solution is injected. Then, behind the palate, 1 to 1½ centimeters within the second molar, or rather, within the border of the gums, 2 mils of the solution are introduced. This type of anesthesia, carried

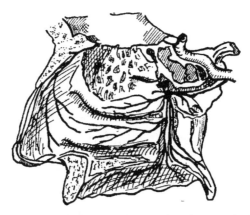

Fig. 49.—To the right are shown the three palatine nerves descending toward the posterior palatine foramen. To the left, at the base of the nose, is the ethmoidal branch of the internal nasal nerve.

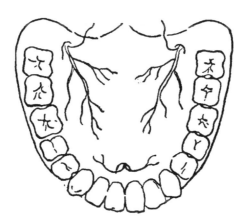

Fig. 50.—Anesthesia of the hard palate. (*Pauchet.*) In front is the nasopalatine nerve, ½ centimeter behind the middle incisors. The surgeon·injects 1 mil of a 2 per cent. solution directly under the mucous membrane. Behind, the nerves emerging from the posterior foramen to the right and left, 1 centimeter within and above the last molar, 1 mil of the strong solution is injected beneath the mucous membrane.

out also on the opposite side, permits the surgeon, with the three points of infiltration, to operate on the mucous membrane of the hard palate and periosteum, though not on the teeth.

Anesthesia of the Buccal Nerve.

This nerve rests upon the tuberosity of the superior maxillary and is distributed over the mucous membrane of the cheek. It is accessible, like the superior dental nerve, by an injection passing along the tuberosity and following a vertical line running from the last upper molar to the last lower molar.

Anesthesia of the Inferior Maxillary Nerve.

As already pointed out, the trunk of the inferior maxillary nerve is accessible, at its emergence from the foramen ovale, by the same route and with the same procedure as was described for infiltration of the Gasserian ganglion. To limit the injection to this trunk, it is sufficient to make the injection upon arriving at but not entering the foramen ovale. The advance of the needle should be arrested as soon as the resistance of the bone ceases, indicating that the anterior border of the aperture has been passed.

The following mode of procedure reaches the nerve without risk of penetrating too far, and the operator should be as familiar with it as with the method first described, as certain conditions may render it preferable, *e.g.,* anatomical deformities, tumors, etc.

The lower border of the zygomatic arch is traced on the skin, its exact center found, and

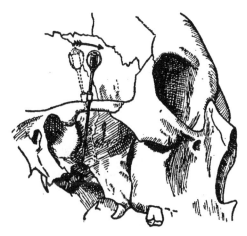

Fig. 51.—Anesthesia of the inferior maxillary nerve. (*Braun.*) The operator places a small fragment of cork upon the needle, as an index. The needle is introduced just below the center of the zygomatic arch. At a depth of 4 centimeters the point touches the pterygoid process. With the needle held firmly in position, the cork is slid down to a level with the skin. The needle is then partly withdrawn and reintroduced at an angle, so as to touch a point 1 centimeter behind the point first reached. When the index cork touches the skin, the point of the needle is near the foramen ovale and when it comes in contact with the nerve the patient feels a sharp pain in the lower jaw. Two mils of a 2 per cent. solution of procaine-adrenin are then injected.

a dermal wheal made at this point. A needle 6 centimeters long is now introduced transversely to a depth of 4 to 5 centimeters so that its point will strike against the pterygoid process, which is 1 centimeter from the foramen ovale. As a guide a thread or small piece of rubber, passed over the

needle before its introduction, is now fastened precisely at a level with the skin. The needle is then
drawn toward the operator, though *not withdrawn
altogether,* and re-inserted to the depth marked on
the needle, aiming, however, about 1 centimeter
behind the bony obstruction (pterygoid). The
earlier and later directions of the needle should

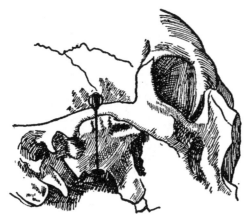

Fig. 52.—Direct injection of the inferior maxillary at the
foramen ovale. (*Braun.*) The needle is introduced at the
junction of the middle and posterior thirds of the zygomatic
arch and directed inward about 5 centimeters, when it will
reach the foramen ovale. If it strikes bone, the latter is the
pterygoid process; it should then be withdrawn a few centimeters and reintroduced further back. The foramen ovale is
located immediately behind the pterygoid process.

form between them an angle of 30°. As soon as
the needle has reached the same depth, though
somewhat posteriorly, it is pushed a few millimeters further in, and the patient will feel a
sharp pain in the tongue or the inferior maxillary.
This indicates that the needle is in the body of
the nerve (Figs. 51, 52). Five mils of a 2 per
cent. procaine-adrenin solution are now injected.

(See also Offerhaus's procedure, p. 98.)

ANESTHESIA OF THE INFERIOR DENTAL NERVE

This is a large terminal branch of the inferior maxillary. It diverges at an acute angle from the lingual nerve and passes between the internal

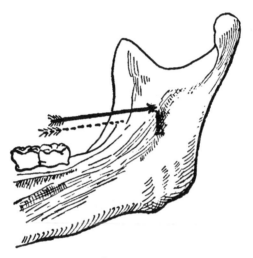

Fig. 53.—Injection of the inferior dental nerve at the inferior dental foramen. (*Braun.*) The arrow indicates the point at which the nerve should be injected. The dotted arrow shows the retromolar trigone. The needle should be first directed to this trigone 1 centimeter above the molar, then should follow the inner wall of the maxillary bone until its point reaches the nerve. One to 2 mils of a 2 per cent. solution are then injected.

pterygoid muscle and the ascending ramus of the inferior maxillary bone until, arriving at the posterior orifice of the dental canal, it emerges on a level with the chin through the mental foramen.

Upon examination of an inferior maxillary bone, there will be found immediately behind the last molar a triangular bony surface, limited externally by a prolongation of the coronoid process and within by a ridge of bone which, likewise detached from the process, passes down toward the inner side of the alveolus of the third molar.

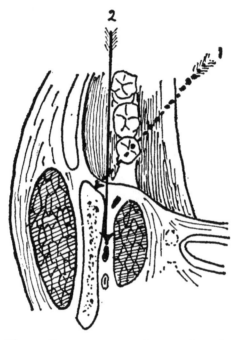

Fig. 54.—Shows the movements imparted to the needle to reach the inferior dental foramen. (*Pauchet.*) The lingual nerve may be reached in the same way.

This small triangle which is normally covered with mucous membrane, serves as the principal landmark in the introduction of the needle.

The patient is seated in front of the operator, with his mouth wide open. The index finger is passed into the mouth, the anterior border of the coronoid found, and within this border the retromolar trigone (Braun) located.   A needle 9 centimeters long is taken in the right hand, and being kept 1 centimeter from the inferior canine on the

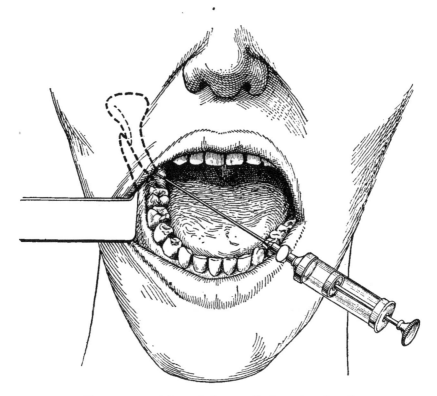

Fig. 55.—First position of the needle in going for the retromolar trigone. (*Pauchet.*) The needle should at first be kept in contact with the canine tooth of the opposite side until the trigone is reached. The handle of the syringe is then swung to the opposite side, so the needle is on a line with the teeth, and pushed along the border of the bone to the foramen.

opposite side, on a level with the grinding surface of the teeth, directed toward the trigone, *i.e.,* the intra-buccal fold of the coronoid.   The point of the needle penetrates the mucous membrane 1 centimeter above and outside of the last molar.

As soon as the membrane has been punctured the point strikes against bone; if not, the point is too far within. Then the operator, feeling his way, inserts the point of the needle until it reaches the ridge of the bone (Fig. 54). It should slide

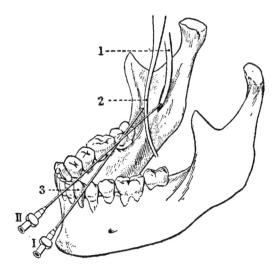

Fig. 56.—Anesthesia of the inferior dental and lingual nerves on the right side. (*Pauchet.*) (1) Right inferior dental nerve. (2) Right lingual nerve. (3) Left inferior canine. The needle is directed from the left lower canine toward the anterior border of the ascending ramus of the right inferior maxillary (Position 1). It is then directed to the internal surface and introduced to a depth of about 2 centimeters (Position II).

along the inner surface of the inferior maxillary; then, without losing its contact with the bone, penetrate 2 to 2½ more centimeters, at which point the operator injects 5 mils of a 1 per cent. solution (Figs. 53, 55, and 56).

Anesthesia of the Mental Nerve.

On a vertical line passing at the same time the supra- and infra- orbital nerves and corresponding to the space between the two first lower molars, is to be found the mental foramen of the inferior maxillary. This is situated at equal distances from the superior and inferior borders of the jaw, and below the interval between the first and second molars. After passing through the soft tissues to this point, the surgeon injects a 2 per cent. solution of procaine-adrenin.

Anesthesia of the Lingual Nerve.

This leaves the inferior dental nerve and branches off to the tongue, describing a curve with an antero-superior concavity. It should be borne in mind that this nerve is in the lower part of the tongue, situated very superficially beneath the mucous membrane.

The procedure is therefore, as follows: The tongue is held in a compress and brought forward toward the opposite corner of the mouth. A line of anesthesia 4 centimeters long is made in the groove formed by the tongue and gums, with a 1 or 2 per cent. solution of procaine-adrenin.

This nerve may also be infiltrated by proceeding as for the inferior dental.

REMARKS.

It would seem, at first sight, that in facial operations, anesthesia of the Gasserian ganglion should prove all sufficient. Actually this is not the case. In the first place, the severity of the Gasserian procedure justifies its employment only in serious interventions, as already pointed out. It is preferable, therefore, to anesthetize the peripheral trunks. Again, there exist anastomoses with the cranial nerves or with branches of the cervical plexus, which would render the anesthesia incomplete were it confined to a single nerve trunk.

Indications for subcutaneous peripheral infiltration, or for the spraying or application of cocaine to the mucous membranes, therefore, frequently exist. These various procedures, trunk anesthesia, local infiltration, and local application, are of mutual assistance and it is a combination of the three which. produces a practically complete anesthesia.

REGIONAL ANESTHESIA IN RHINOLOGY.

SUBMUCOUS RESECTION OF THE CARTILAGE OF THE NASAL SEPTUM.

Tampons of a strong solution of adrenin-cocaine are applied for 10 minutes. A 2 per cent. solution of procaine-adrenin is injected under the mucous membrane of the septum, both on its convex and its concave surfaces. One should infiltrate also, especially if the deviation is extensive, the three nerve trunks which together sensitize the septum, above and forward, below and forward, in the floor and behind.

HYPERTROPHY OF THE LOWER AND MIDDLE TURBINATES.

Resection of the Upper and Lower Turbinates and of Nasal Myxomas.—Tampons of cocaine which contract the mucous membrane usually suf-

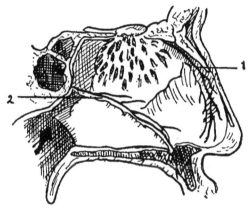

Fig. 57.—(1) Ethmoidal branch of the internal nasal nerve. (2) Nasopalatine nerve which supplies the wall and emerges through the anterior palatine foramen, behind the incisors. (*Pauchet.*)

fice. In the case of the upper turbinate, however, their use is disadvantageous because it diminishes the already small area concerned. It is preferable, therefore, to infiltrate the affected tissues, as this augments their volume. In the presence of numerous polypi, tamponing is tedious and sometimes impossible. We therefore inject the ethmoidal, nasal, and septal nerves, thus rendering the parts anesthetic (Fig. 57).

Moure's Operation for Large Tumors of the Brain.

(*a*) Application of cocaine tampons to the olfactory mucosa; (*b*) infiltration of the ethmoidal

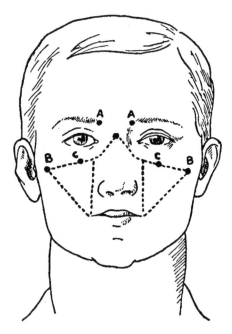

Fig. 58.—Operation of Moure. Resection of the ethmoid after having displaced downward the ascending branch of the superior maxillary and enlarged the anterior orifice of the bones of the nasal fossa without regard to the superior maxillary. (*A*) Infiltration of the ethmoidal nerve by the internal orbital route. (*B*) Infiltration of the superior maxillary nerve (see Figs. 43 and 44). (*C*) Emergence of the infraorbital nerve.

nerves; (*c*) infiltration of the superior maxillary nerve; (*d*) infiltration of the infraorbital nerve; (*e*) infiltration of a line from the corner of the mouth upward, as shown in Fig. 58. Peripheral infiltration following a broken line uniting the corner of the mouth with the junction of the superior maxillary nerve and the base of the nasal lobe.

INJECTION OF THE MAXILLARY SINUS (LUC'S OPERATION.)

(a) Tamponing the nasal cavity with gauze soaked with cocaine; (b) infiltration of the eth-

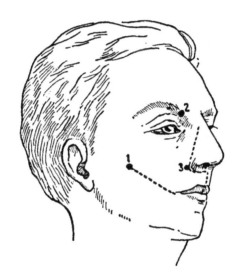

Fig. 59.—Trephining the maxillary sinus. (*Labouré.*) (1) Infiltration of the superior maxillary nerve at the foramen ovale (Figs. 43 and 44). (2) Anesthesia of the ethmoidal nerve by the internal orbital route (Fig. 41). The subcutaneous infiltration is shown by the dotted lines.

moidal and superior maxillary nerves; (c) infiltration through the mouth of the canine fossa and the region of the infraorbital nerve (Fig. 59).

Injection of the Frontal Sinus.

(*a*) Tamponing the anterior superior nasal fossa with gauze soaked with cocaine; (*b*) infiltration of the superior maxillary nerve; (*c*) infil-

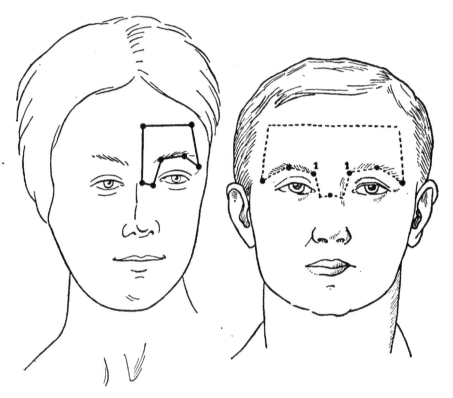

Figs. 60, 61.—Trephining the frontal sinus, one side and both sides. (*Pauchet.*) (1) Internal orbital injection (Fig. 41). (2) Point of injection for the superior maxillary nerve (Figs. 43 and 44). Through the several dermal wheals, the field of operation is circumscribed along the dotted lines.

tration of the ethmoidal nerves; (*d*) subcutaneous and preperiosteal injections surrounding the operative field (Figs. 60, 61).

Operations upon the Sphenoidal Sinuses and for Sarcoma of the Hypophysis.

The endonasal route is followed; submucous resection of the cartilaginous and bony septum; infiltration of both sides of the septum and of the ethmoidal nerves.

REGIONAL ANESTHESIA IN OTOLOGY.

Nerve Supply.

The middle ear receives its sensory supply from Jacobson's nerve, a branch of the glossopharyngeal, and the superficial petrosal nerve.

The tympanum and external auditory canal are supplied by two nerves, which enter, the one anteriorly, the other posteriorly. The anterior is the auriculo-temporal nerve, a branch of the superior maxillary, which supplies the antero-inferior floor of the external canal. The posterior nerve is the auricular branch of the pneumogastric. These nerves enter the canal at the union of its cartilaginous and osseous portions.

The external ear is supplied by the great auricular nerve, the auriculo-temporal, the lesser occipital, and the auricular branch of the pneumogastric.

The nerve supply of the mastoid region consists of the sub-occipital and the superior cervical nerves, through branches from the mastoid.

All of these nerve branches intercommunicate, and practically their respective limits are hard to define.

Technique.

Anesthesia of the Middle Ear and Tympanum.
—In the middle ear the nerves are superficial and
sub-mucous, and can be desensitized with Bonain's
solution:

℞ Cocaine hydrochloride,
   Menthol,
   Phenol .... āā 1 grain.
   Adrenin .... 0.001 grain.

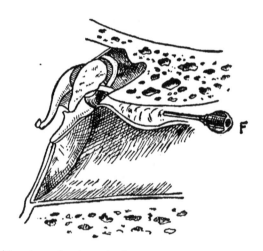

Fig. 62.—Anesthesia of the auditory canal. (*Labouré.*)
The needle is introduced at the junction of the cartilage and
bone on the superior and posterior walls. When it has penetrated 2 millimeters, a 2 per cent. solution is injected.

Upon application of this agent one may painlessly curette vegetations, remove a polyp, or
puncture the tympanic membrane.

For more severe procedures, such as ossiculectomy, the external auditory canal is anesthetized
by the following procedure (Neumann) (Fig. 62):

A large speculum is passed into the canal and inclined backward or laterally, thus bringing into view the point of junction of the cartilage with the bone. At this point, above and behind, at the junction of superior and posterior walls, a needle is inserted for 2 millimeters, a few drops of solution slowly injected, and a bony contact felt for. The bone, when reached, should be followed for some distance in order to make certain of injecting the remainder of the solution into the subperiosteal zone. Such an injection anesthetizes the upper portion of the tympanum, the vestibule, and the ossicles. One should wait 10 minutes before operating.

The injection just described acts in the following manner: On a level with Schrapnel's membrane, the two epithelial linings meet, the fibrous tissue of the tympanum being wanting. An injection of fluid following the epithelium of the canal penetrates under the epithelium of the middle ear on a level with the flaccid membrane and ascends under the mucous membrane that lines the vestibule, since it is at no time arrested by any barrier (Molinar[1]).

Anesthesia of the External Auditory Canal.— The external auditory canal is supplied by two nerves which penetrate in front and behind, at the union of the cartilaginous and bony portions of the canal. They can be reached either through the canal or from behind the auricle.

---

[1] Adolph Molinar: "Regional Anesthesia for Operations upon the Auditory Apparatus."

The needle is directed backward toward the
tympano-mastoid fissure in the direction of the
pneumogastric. Procaine-adrenin solution is injected while introducing the needle. Then the
latter is withdrawn 1 centimeter, without entirely
removing it, directed downward, forward, and inward toward the condyle of the maxillary, and

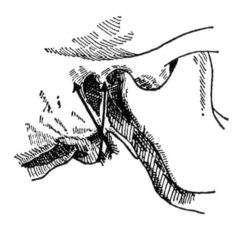

Fig. 63.—Showing a V-shaped injection, in its
relations to the bony parts.

during the course of this movement, 2 mils of
procaine-adrenin solution injected to a depth of
not more than 2 centimeters. After this procedure, operations for furuncles or exostosis in the
canal can be satisfactorily carried out (Fig. 63).

*Anesthesia of the External Ear and Mastoid
Region.*—Encircle the external ear and mastoid
region with a series of injections which cross each
other in the superficial and deep tissues (Fig. 64).

It is useless to try to penetrate beneath the
periosteum; its close adhesion renders this impos-

sible. Besides, such a procedure would be unnecessary. The bone receives its nerve supply from without, *i.e.,* from the scalp. The operator may, if he so desires, inject along the line of the proposed incision.

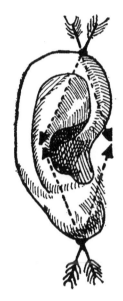

Fig. 64.—Anesthesia of the external ear. (*Labouré.*)
Two wheals, superior and inferior, are made and injections executed in the direction of the arrows, describing a diamond-shaped figure about the ear.

These various forms of anesthesia, viz., the application of 'Bonain's mixture to the tympanum or vestibule; infiltration of the vestibule through the canal; infiltration of the auriculo-temporal nerves and the auricular branch of the pneumogastric; peripheral anesthesia around the external ear and mastoid, constitute a series of procedures necessary and sufficient for a number of different oper-

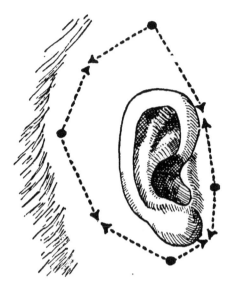

Fig. 65.—Mastoidectomy.   (*Labouré.*)   A subcutaneous polygon is infiltrated through four wheals, the needle entering in the direction of the arrows.

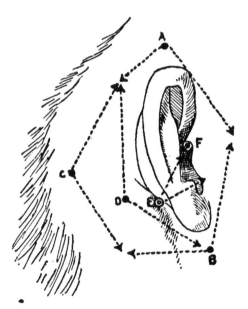

Fig. 66.—Petromastoid operation. (*Labouré.*) After having infiltrated as in Fig. 65, three more wheals are made and injections executed in the direction of the two arrows (*D*) and the arrows (*E* and *F*).

ations.   One may employ one procedure, or another, or all procedures combined, according to the case.

In general, the relative indications for each may be -stated thus: 1. For perforation of the tympanum: Application of Bonain's mixture, which drives the blood from the tissues and indicates to the operator the area anesthetized.   2. For ossiculectomy: Infiltration of the superior wall of the canal and vestibule, and application of Bonain's mixture.   3. For furuncle of the canal: Infiltration of the anterior and posterior nerves by an injection through the auriculo-mastoid sulcus. 4. For plastic operations on the external ear: Peripheral anesthesia in circular form instituted around the external ear as a center.   5. For mastoiditis: As in the preceding (Figs. 65, 66).   6. For curettage: A combination of all the preceding methods.

REGIONAL ANESTHESIA IN OPHTHALMOLOGY.

Nerve Supply.

The orbit and ocular globe receive their nerve supply from the branches of the ophthalmic.   In addition, the orbital branch of the superior maxillary supplies, through its terminal trunks—the temporo-malar nerves,—the skin of the temple, of the malar region, and about the external angle of the eye (Figs. 37, 38, 39).

Technique.

Anesthesia of the ophthalmic nerve and its branches may be obtained by external and internal orbital injections, the technique of which has already been described (Figs. 40, 41, 42, with several pages describing the ophthalmic and its branches).

If necessary the anesthesia may be completed by infiltration of the superior maxillary nerve or of a few of its branches, as already described under Anesthesia of the Superior Maxillary.

For completion of the anesthesia in respect of the ciliary nerves or the ciliary ganglion, the muscular pyramid which immediately surrounds the ocular globe should be infiltrated. In order to effect this, one should direct the needle toward the vault of the orbit, keeping as close as possible to the outer surface of the eye-ball. Five mils of a 1 per cent. procaine-adrenin solution are injected, and the sub-conjunctival tissue also infiltrated. A needle is introduced into the external commissure of the eyelids, and pushed down between the conjunctiva and the bulb. Then, a little to the inside, at a depth of 4½ centimeters, *i.e.,* close to the ciliary ganglion, 1 mil of a 2 per cent. solution is injected. Finally ½ mil of this strong solution is injected under the conjunctiva surrounding the bulb. Thus, whatever be the operation,—enucleation, etc.,—perfect anesthesia will be obtained.

Operations on the Eyelids and Lachrymal Gland (Fig. 67).—A few drops of cocaine on the conjunctiva, together with an injection of 2 mils of a ½ per cent. solution of procaine-adrenin near the superior bony wall, will anesthetize the upper eyelid.

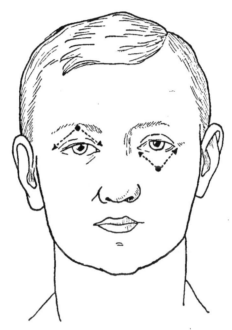

Fig. 67.—Anesthesia of the eyelids. (*Pauchet.*) One injection through a wheal suffices for each eyelid.

For the lower eyelid, one should inject 2 mils along the inferior orbital wall, in a fan-shaped area 2 centimeters deep and 2 across. The infra-orbital nerve, and the anterior ethmoidal, which supplies the internal portion of the lower eyelid, are infiltrated.

Cataract; Iridectomy.—(*a*) Drop a few drops of a $\frac{1}{20}$ per cent. solution onto the eyeball, several times, as it will then act by absorption. (*b*) Inject ½ mil of ½ per cent. solution procaine-adrenin under the conjunctiva.

Enucleation of the Eyeball.—(*a*) Inject 2 or 3 mils of solution through the external superior angle. (*b*) Repeat this procedure at the internal angle. (*c*) Infiltrate the superior maxillary nerve either through the orbit or the malar region.

REGIONAL ANESTHESIA IN DENTAL SURGERY.

Nerve Supply

As regards the upper teeth, the nerves first follow above the outer side of the tuberosity of the superior maxillary, then penetrate it in order to reach the dental pulp. Here they are distributed also to the periosteum, the mucous membrane, and the alveolar tissue.

The lower teeth are supplied by the inferior dental nerve, which enters the inferior maxillary bone at the inferior dental foramen and forms the inferior dental plexus, then divides into two branches, one in the bone,—the incisor, which supplies the incisor teeth,—the other, the mental, which supplies the chin and lower lip. The lower gums and tongue are supplied by the lingual nerve. The region of the incisors is supplied by branches coming from the inferior dental, mental, and lingual nerves, all more or less inter-related.

TECHNIQUE.

Infiltration of the Dental Branches in the Upper Jaw.—A ½ per cent solution is used. From 2 to 10 mils suffices, according to whether it is desired to anesthetize one tooth or an entire half of the jaw. As the dental branches lie superficially, immediately under the mucous membrane in the fold of the gum, the injection is readily carried out and its result immediate. The point of injection varies according to the teeth to be rendered anesthetic:

(*a*) For the *incisors,* one should infiltrate the submucous membrane in the median line, either on the level of the frænum linguæ or on the nasal floor near the septum, or at both of these points.

(*b*) For the *canine* and *first molars,* the injection is made above the canine tooth.

(*c*) For the *large molars,* one infiltrates well back at the outer border of the tuberosity of the maxillary, and even at its posterior border if a curved needle is available. Again, it may be considered necessary to enter through the cheek, to a depth of 2½ centimeters, in the direction of the superior maxillary nerve.

To permit of convenient infiltration, an aid should draw aside the labial commissures with small retractors.

Where the work bears on half the maxillary arch, infiltration should be carried out along its entire length.

On principle, one should not infiltrate the trunk of the superior maxillary nerve. Yet there need be no hesitation in doing so in cases of severe buccal septicemia.

Infiltration of the Lower Teeth.—Where the incisors and canine teeth are concerned, one may proceed as for the upper jaw, infiltrating the submucous membrane in order to reach the ramifications of the mental and incisor nerves.

For the remaining lower teeth this procedure is insufficient because the inferior dental nerve lies in the center of the maxillary bone, which is very thick at this point. One should, therefore, infiltrate the trunk of the nerve at the dental foramen as already described. The labial commissure is retracted, the ascending branch of the inferior maxillary nerve found, and 3 to 5 mils of a ½ per cent. solution of procaine injected into its center. (Figs. 55 and 56.)

If the buccal cavity is too septic, the inferior dental nerve can be anesthetized from the outside; or 2 mils of anesthetic solution may be injected under the dental collar of the last molars in order to infiltrate the gingival branches of the buccinator—which, however, are not very large.

Unilateral injections under the gums for the lower incisors are insufficient because of the anastomoses of the two incisor nerves. To obtain complete insensibility, both nerves must be infiltrated even for an operation involving only one side. Two mils of solution are injected on each side of the median line; at this point there is a slight depression, the thin, grooved wall of which permits of absorption of the procaine.

REGIONAL ANESTHESIA OF THE FACE AND JAWS.

The soft tissues of the face are supplied by the three branches of the trigeminus, the ramifica-

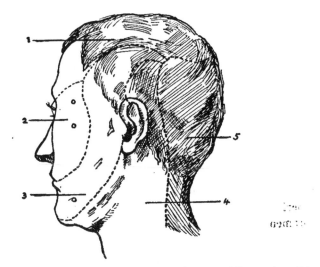

Fig. 68.—The sensory areas of the head. (*Testut.*) (1) Ophthalmic. (2) Superior maxillary. (3) Inferior maxillary. (4) Cervical plexus (anterior branches). (5) Cervical plexus (posterior branches).

tions of which are so intermingled as to render trunk infiltration insufficient for complete anesthesia. Even infiltration of the Gasserian ganglion of one side yields only an incomplete anesthesia when the operative procedure is conducted near the median line.

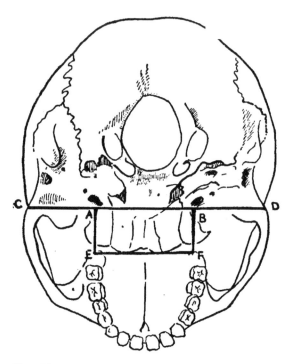

Fig. 69.—The measurements of Offerhaus. The "tubercle
line" *C D* passes a few millimeters in front of and below the
foramen ovale at points *A* and *B*. The distance *E F* from one
superior dental arch to the other, is equal to *A B* from one
foramen ovale to the other. Measuring C *D* and *E F*, sub-
tracting the latter from the former, and dividing the result by
2 yields the distance C *A* or *D B*. This procedure constitutes
an alternative method for injecting the superior maxillary
nerve at the foramen ovale. (*Cf.* pp. 72-74.)

ANESTHESIA OF THE MIDFRONTAL REGION.

The frontal zone is supplied by branches of the
ophthalmic nerve,—lachrymal, frontal, and nasal,—
which ascend from below. It is sufficient, therefore, to institute a horizontal line of infiltration,
both intradermal and subperiosteal, passing above
the convexity of the two eyebrows (Fig. 40).

ANESTHESIA OF THE NOSE, LIPS, AND CHEEKS.

The lobe of the nose is easily rendered insensible by means of a circular infiltration outlining its base (Figs. 70 and 71). Thus, in the case of a tumor of the lobe requiring surgical intervention, four injections should be made through

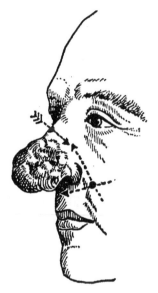

Fig. 70.—Circumscribing the lobe of the nose. (*Braun.*)

dermal wheals located as follows: One on the bridge of the nose, two at the base of the alæ, and the fourth at the base of the nasal septum on the upper lip.

The upper lip (Fig. 71) may be desensitized by three lines: One transversal, going from the base of one ala to the other, and the two others vertical, descending from the extremities of the preceding points to the labial commissures and also

ascending to meet at the bridge of the nose. Two
bands. of infiltration should thus be made, the one
subcutaneous, the other submucous, the needle being directed parallel with the mucous membrane
by means of a gloved finger introduced under the
lip.

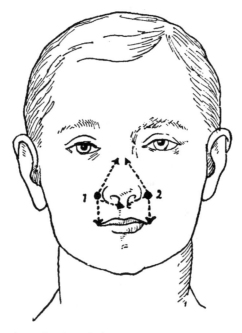

Fig. 71.—Anesthesia of the lobe of the nose and the upper
lip through two wheals, following the direction of the arrows.
(*Pauchet.*)

Infiltration of the upper lip may usually be
combined with that for the lobe of the nose.
The anesthetized area may be enlarged at will according to the necessities of the operation (as in
the pentagon, Fig. 72).

For harelip one should infiltrate a band extending from the commissure of the lips to the

infraorbital foramen, connected by a transverse line across the dorsum nasi.

The anemia produced by the adrenin facilitates operative work. The tissues are not altered by peripheral infiltration made at a distance.

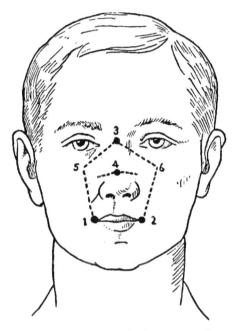

Fig. 72.—Anesthesia for facial operations (*Pauchet.*) There are two median wheals, central and superior, and two lateral and inferior wheals. (5) and (6) serve for anesthesia of the infraorbital nerve. (4) applies in anesthesia of the ethmoidal nerve. The dotted polygon is a line of infiltration made with a 1 per cent. solution.

For the lower lip a single dermal wheal should be made on the chin, and from this point two divergent lines of infiltration made both under the skin and under the mucous membrane, with the needle guided by a finger introduced in the mouth. The chin and subjacent *symphysis menti* some-

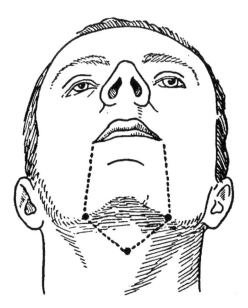

Fig. 73.—Median section of the body of the inferior maxillary. (*Pauchet.*) The anterior and posterior sections of the body of the maxillary bone are infiltrated through three wheals.

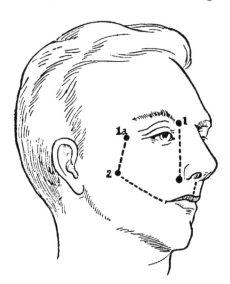

Fig. 74.—Anesthesia for resection of the superior maxillary bone. (1) and (1a) External and internal orbital injections. (2) Injection of the superior maxillary nerve. A weak procaine-adrenin solution is used in instituting the subcutaneous bands of infiltration.

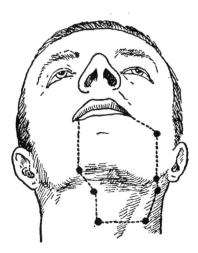

Fig. 75.—Unilateral resection of the lower jaw (*Pauchet.*) The inferior dental nerve is injected at the inferior dental foramen, or the inferior maxillary nerve at the foramen ovale, and the subcutaneous tissue then infiltrated along the dotted line.

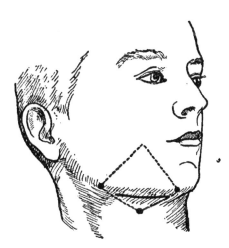

Fig. 76.—Operation on the horizontal portion of the lower maxillary bone. (*Pauchet.*) The inferior dental nerve is anesthetized at the inferior dental foramen or the inferior maxillary nerve at the foramen ovale, and a subcutaneous diamond-shaped figure infiltrated through three wheals. The dark line indicates the incision.

times require to be rendered insensible, *e.g.,* for the suture of a fracture of the mandible (Fig. 73):

(1) A horse-shoe-shaped band of infiltration following the lower border of the inferior maxillary bone, both subcutaneous and subperiosteal.

(2) Infiltration of the mental nerve on one, or better both sides, even if the operation be unilateral.

Resection of the Superior Maxillary (Fig. 74). —If the lesion is extensive and likely to cause the surgeon to go beyond the superior maxillary, he is justified in infiltrating the Gasserian ganglion, as already explained. Generally, however, it proves sufficient to proceed thus: (1) Infiltrate the superior maxillary nerve. (2) Infiltrate the inferior maxillary nerve. (3) Infiltrate the orbital nerves by two injections in the superior-internal and superior-external angles. (4) Infiltrate the hard and soft palates, following the line of incision.

For the lower jaw (Figs. 75 and 76) the inferior maxillary nerve should be infiltrated at the foramen ovale or at the dental foramen with a ½ per cent. solution and the field of operation circumscribed with peripheral injections of a 1 per cent. solution. One can then operate on the bone for suturing or resection. In the event of cancer at the alveolar border, the nerves should be infiltrated at the inferior dental foramen. For disarticulation of the jaw the foramen ovale should be infiltrated.

REGIONAL ANESTHESIA OF THE TONGUE, FLOOR OF THE MOUTH, TONSILS, AND PALATE.

NERVE SUPPLY.

The lingual nerve supplies two-thirds of the anterior portion of the tongue and the floor of the mouth; the glosso-pharyngeal nerve supplies the posterior portion of the tongue, the region of

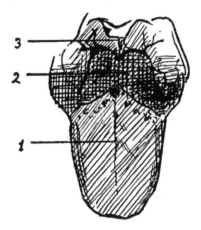

Fig. 77.—Sensory distributions on the tongue. (*Testut.*) (1) Lingual. (2) Glossopharyngeal. (3) Superior laryngeal.

the tonsils, and the pharynx; the superior maxillary nerve supplies the soft palate and the anterior pillars of the fauces, and the superior laryngeal nerve supplies the epiglottis.

One may therefore infiltrate the following trunks:

(1) The lingual nerve, within the inferior dental foramen, desensitizing two-thirds of the anterior portion of the tongue and the floor of the mouth.

(2) The superior laryngeal nerve, in the thyro-hyoid space (see page 116).

(3) Infiltration of the glosso-pharyngeal and pneumogastric nerves should be avoided because it is dangerous; peripheral infiltration must be substituted.

TECHNIQUE.

Excision of a Tumor of the Margin of the Tongue.—A triangle enclosing the tumor is out-

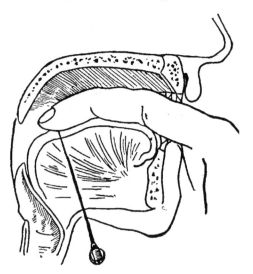

Fig. 78.—Anesthesia of the tongue and the buccal floor. (*Pauchet.*) With a finger placed over the base of the tongue the needle is introduced above the hyoid bone until its point almost touches the finger on the tongue, coming to rest just beneath the mucous membrane.

lined by two V-shaped bands of infiltration. The growth can then be excised without hemorrhage or pain.

Excision of an Extensive Cancer or Large Cyst of the Floor of the Mouth.—A long needle is introduced under the chin, above the hyoid bone, and pushed in vertically toward the base of the tongue, being received against the tip of the left index finger, introduced into the mouth as for tracheotomy. This vertical route is first infiltrated, then through the same wheal one injects successively from top to bottom and further and further out, as many layers as are necessary to form a fan shaped infiltrated region, the sides of which extend to the maxillary bones, thus blocking off

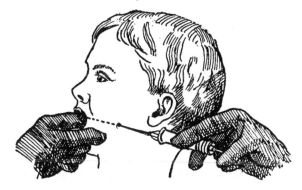

Fig. 79.—Injection for transverse incision of the cheek for cancer of the pharynx or posterior cancer of the tongue. (*Pauchet.*)

all the nerves of the anterior portion of the tongue.

Restricted Operations on the Floor of the Mouth. —Small tumors of the floor of the mouth may be infiltrated in a circle, by an injection made from under the chin, with the needle always guided by the finger in the mouth.

Removal of Extensive Cancer of the Tongue, Floor of the Mouth, and Tonsils.—(1) The two inferior maxillary nerves are infiltrated at the inferior dental foramen: (2) the base of the tongue is infiltrated by a subhyoid injection; (3) peripheral infiltration of the operative field is insti-

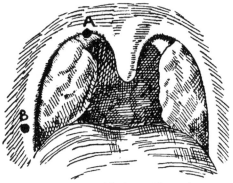

Fig. 80.—Tonsillectomy (*Labouré.*) The superior pole is infiltrated by an injection made in the upper part of the anterior pillar. An injection at the base of this pillar infiltrates the inferior pole. Quinine is employed.

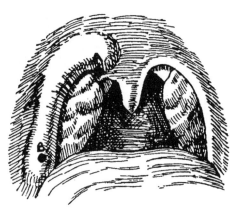

Fig. 81.—Tonsillectomy. (*Labouré.*) The inferior pillar is completely infiltrated. Quinine infiltration of the tonsil has been instituted (white crescent)

tuted; (4) in some cases the Gasserian ganglion of one side is also infiltrated.

Operations on the Palate.—Anesthesia of both the soft and hard palate may be obtained by making an injection under the mucous membrane inside of the large molars and behind the middle incisors. For resection of the bony hard palate, the two superior maxillary nerves should be infiltrated.

In staphylorrhaphies one should avoid using too much adrenin at the point where the flaps are to be made.

Tonsillectomy (Figs. 80 and 81).—Infiltrate the two nerve pedicles of the tonsil: (1) At the lower portion of the anterior pillar; (2) at the upper part of the vestibule, at the junction of the posterior and anterior pillars.

REGIONAL ANESTHESIA IN OPERATIONS ON THE NECK.

INFILTRATION OF THE CERVICAL ROOTS.

The soft tissues of the anterior portion of the neck are supplied by the anterior branches of the 2d, 3d, and 4th cervical nerves, of which the terminal branches—*auricular, mastoid, transverse cervical,* and *supraclavicular,*—emerge at the posterior margin of the sterno-mastoid muscle (Fig. 82).

Infiltration of these terminal branches at the posterior border of the sterno-cleido-mastoid desensitizes the skin alone and this is rarely sufficient. In order to obtain a deep anesthesia, the nerves must be reached at their emergence from the spinal column, on a level with the transverse processes of the 3d, 4th, and 5th vertebræ (Fig. 86).

The distribution of the cervical trunks is as follows (see Figs. 85 and 87): The second cervical supplies the nape of the neck and the occipital region. The third cervical supplies the antero-

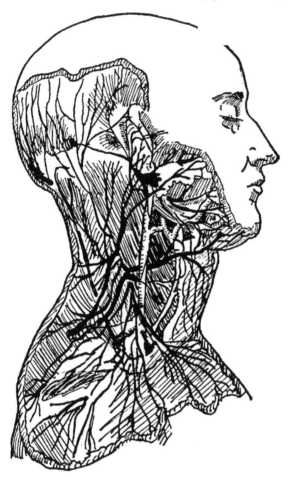

Fig. 82.—Superficial branches of the cervical plexus (*Hirschfeld.*) These branches should be desensitized by infiltration of the soft tissues lying between the mastoid and the upper margin of the cricoid cartilage, following a vertical line and injecting through 3 wheals.

lateral portions of the neck, from the lower jaw to the shoulders and the upper portions of the arms. The roots of the second, third, and fourth cervical supply the cervical plexus (see Figs. 83 to 85). It is these roots, therefore, that must be reached in operating on the neck.

Technique.—The line of skin infiltration for the cervical ·plexus is vertical, *i.e.,* parallel with

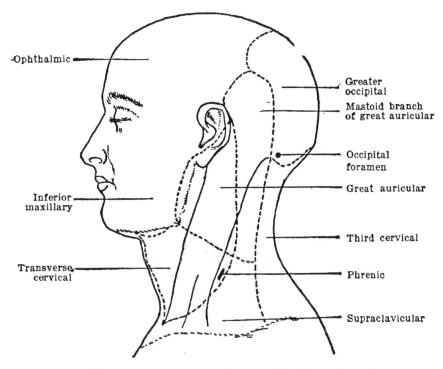

Fig. 83.—Sensory areas of the superficial branches of the cervical plexus. (*Testut.*)

the spinal column, and is determined by the two following points: Above, a point one finger-breadth below the tip of the mastoid, corresponding to the angle of the jaw; below, a point 5 centimeters lower down and corresponding to the superior border of the thyroid cartilage. Using a 6-centimeter needle, the bone should be encoun-

tered at a depth of 5 centimeters, and a fan-
shaped injection of a 1 per cent. solution of procaine-adrenin made there. About 25 mils is sufficient. The needle should be introduced through

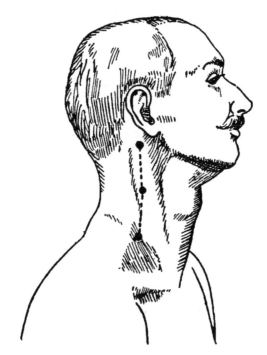

Fig. 84.—Anesthesia of the cervical plexus. (*Pauchet.*)
On a line joining the mastoid and the tubercle of the 6th cervical transverse process (1 to 3) a layer of soft tissues, extending from the skin to the spinal column and from the
lower border of the inferior maxillary (1) to a point situated
on a level with the cricoid (2), is infiltrated.

the wheals indicated and the fluid injected as it
is withdrawn. There is thus infiltrated an area
about 5 centimeters square, outlined on the skin
by the preceding line, above and below by a perpendicular line passing from these points to the
vertebral column, and involving the tissues bor-

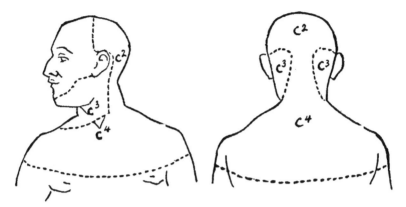

Fig. 85.—Anesthesia resulting from paravertebral injection of the cervical plexus (anterolateral and posterior view). (*Testut.*)

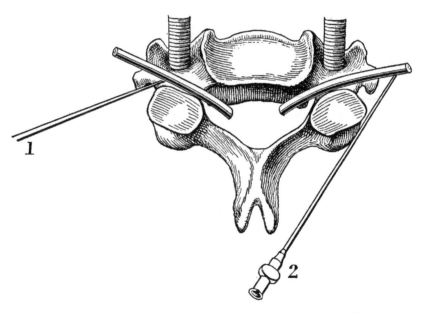

Fig. 86.—Paravertebral anesthesia of the neck. (*Danys.*) Needle (1) is aimed directly at the lateral portion of the vertebra, but it almost touches the vertebral artery. Needle (2) (Danys) enters 2 centimeters from the spinous process, comes in contact with the lateral mass of the vertebra, and reaches the nerve without danger to the vertebral artery.

8

dering the column between the two perpendicular
lines (Fig. 84).

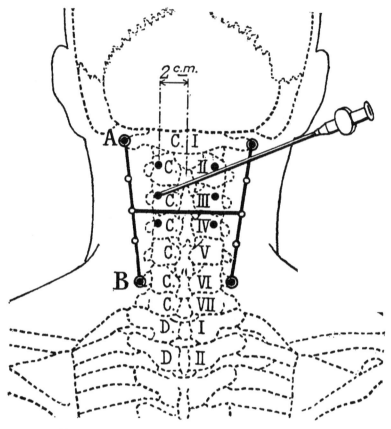

Fig. 87.—Paravertebral anesthesia of the neck. (*Pauchet.*)
A B extends from the mastoid to the 6th cervical vertebra.
The white and black dots indicate the dermal wheals. Along
this line the needle enters transversely to infiltrate the nerve
(direct route). The figure shows the needle penetrating obliquely (*Danys*) 2 centimeters beyond the spinous process and
following the lateral masses of the vertebræ. As soon as it
has passed these a strong solution of procaine-adrenin is
injected.

Danys advises that the needle be introduced
through the posterior surface of the neck, 2 centimeters from the interspinous line, in order to avoid

a possible penetration of the needle into the inter-transverse space and a consequent wounding of the vertebral artery. We prefer, however, the method described above, care being taken not to penetrate too deeply.

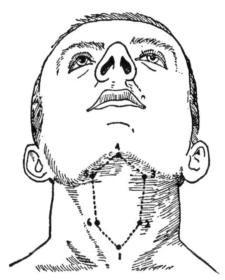

Fig. 88.—Peripheral infiltration for laryngectomy or laryngotomy, circumscribing the larynx. (*Labouré*.) The wheals here shown should be joined by subcutaneous and subfascial bands of infiltration. The wheal corresponding to the thyro-hyoid space is missing from the polygon. Infiltration of the two superior laryngeal nerves through the thyro-hyoid membrane is sufficient.

ANESTHESIA OF THE LARYNGEAL NERVE TRUNKS.

Two nerves supply the larynx,—the superior laryngeal, and the inferior or recurrent laryngeal. The latter is almost exclusively motor, whereas the first is entirely sensory (Fig. 88).

Infiltration of the Superior Laryngeal Nerve.

The superior laryngeal arises from the inferior pole of the plexiform ganglion. It is held against the pharynx by the internal carotid, then by the beginning of the facial and lingual arteries, Slightly above the greater cornu of the hyoid bone it divides into its two terminal branches:

(1) The *superior branch* (*external laryngeal*) follows the vertical insertion of the inferior constrictor over the thyroid gland to the crico-thyroid muscle, which it supplies, and terminates in the subglottic portion of the mucous membrane of the larynx.

(2) The *inferior branch* (*internal laryngeal*) continues in the direction of the common trunk, passes between the thyroid muscle and the hyothyroid membrane, penetrating through the middle of this membrane, and divides into superior terminal filaments for the epiglottis and base of the tongue, inferior filaments for the mucous membrane of the larynx and the arytenoids, and an anastomotic termination for the recurrent nerve (ansa Gallieni).

Technique.—The sensory innervation of the larynx is constituted almost entirely,—above the vocal cords at any rate,—by the superior laryngeal. As already stated, this nerve penetrates immediately behind the posterior extremity of the greater cornu of the hyoid bone, under the inferior border of this bone. It follows closely the thyro-hyoid membrane, courses forward, perforates this membrane, and supplies the laryngeal mucous membrane and the neighboring portions of the pharynx. A needle 6 centimeters long is introduced in the median line between the thyroid cartilage and the hyoid bone, into the thyroid ligament. Once it is in this ligament, the needle is made to approach the greater cornu of the hyoid bone, which is easily felt with the finger. This ligament is now infiltrated on both sides, to the right and to the left, with 5 to 10 mils of a 1 per cent. procaine-adrenin solution.

Infiltration of the Recurrent Laryngeal Nerve. —Even if this nerve were exclusively motor, its infiltration would be justified to avoid spasm of the larynx, but actually it is a mixed nerve. Couzard and Chevrier infiltrate it thus: "Introduce a straight needle into the angle formed in the median line by the superior border of the thyroid, injecting obliquely below, behind, and outside of the angle; come into contact with the internal face of the thyroid cartilage; guide the needle diagonally toward the postero-inferior angle of this cartilage, and inject the solution; it will distend the recess and bathe the terminal branches of the recurrent nerve." One to 2 mils of solution suffices.

These infiltrations of the trunks do not render local anesthesia unnecessary. Spraying with a 20 per cent. solution of cocaine, tamponage with a 10 per cent. solution, and submucous injection of 1 per cent. procaine-adrenin, are all advantageous adjuncts.

OPERATIONS.

(1) *Endolaryngeal Intervention.*—(*a*) One should first anesthetize by spraying and tamponing with a 10 to 20 per cent. solution of cocaine the base of the tongue, the pillars of the fauces and the larynx.

(*b*) Infiltration of the two superior laryngeal nerves should be carried out.

(2) *Tracheotomy, Laryngo-fissure, and Laryngostomy.*—The methods of anesthesia described above should be employed, and intradermal and subcutaneous, peripheral, and trunk anesthesia added. In cases of laryngo-fissure and laryngostomy, as soon as the larynx is open, one may apply tampons moistened with a strong solution of cocaine to the mucous membrane.

(3) *Laryngectomy and Goiter Operations.*—These are more extensive procedures, for the performance of which it is necessary to infiltrate the trunks of the nerves of the plexus and the larynx, and to institute a subcutaneous peripheral infiltration surrounding the larynx or the tumor at a distance.

The harmful actions of chloroform or ether upon the heart, lungs, and liver are thus avoided, to the great benefit of patients whose respiration is affected by disease or who are diabetic. Again, regional anesthesia permits the patient to clear his bronchi during the course of the operation, thus avoiding broncho-pneumonia. Shock is also considerably diminished.

(4) *Ligation of the External Carotid or Thyroid Arteries.*—The cervical plexus is first infiltrated, and there is then circumscribed under the skin and fascia a quadrilateral area extending beyond .the limits of the incision.

(5) *Removal of Enlarged Glands and Tumors of the Neck.*—The cervical plexus of one or both

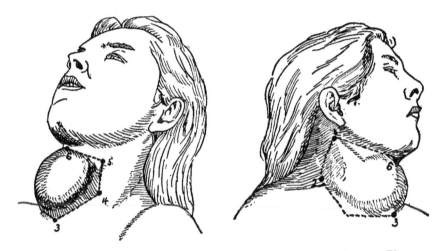

Fig. 89.—Infiltration for thyroidectomy. (*Pauchet.*) The injection to the right infiltrates the branches of the cervical plexus along the transverse processes of the vertebræ (from 1 to 2). The mass is surrounded at a distance with a subcutaneous and subfascial band of infiltration (2, 3, 4, 5, and 6). We have performed about 250 strumectomies by Kocher's method without mortality.

sides is infiltrated and the tumor or lymphatic mass circumscribed by peripheral injection of a ½ per cent. procaine-adrenin solution. If the mass of the tumor or lymphatics extends posteriorly so as to interfere with the passage of the needle,

the latter may, instead of being introduced transversely or in front, be passed in near the interspinous line, in an anterior or in any intermediate
oblique direction.

(6) *Infrahyoid and Suprahyoid Pharyngotomy.*
—The thyroid membrane is infiltrated and a peri-

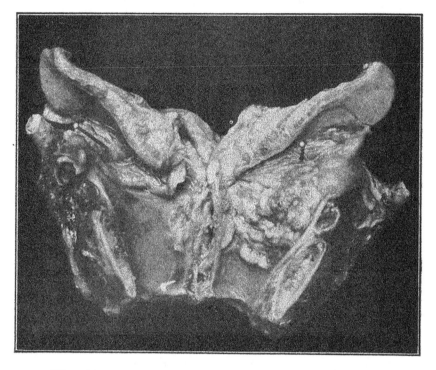

Fig. 90.—Removal of carcinoma of the larynx under
regional anesthesia. (*Pauchet.*) The organ has been opened
up posteriorly; the tumor is to be seen on the right vocal cords.

pheral lozenge-shaped area of infiltration made
over the inferior maxillary and the thyroid cartilage. During the course of the operation it is
sometimes necessary to infiltrate the tumor over
its entire external surface.

(7) *Thyroidectomy.*—Six dermal wheals are made (Figs. 89 and 90). Points 1 and 2 correspond to the line of the transverse processes and serve as landmarks in instituting paravertebral anesthesia of the neck. All the tissues, epidermis, muscles, and nerves are thus infiltrated until the cervical plexus is reached.

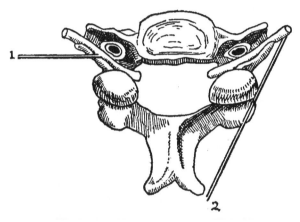

Fig. 91.—Paravertebral anesthesia of the neck. (*Danys.*) This figure shows the two methods of reaching the nerve as it emerges from the spinal canal. Needle 1 aims transversely for the nerve, but it runs a risk of injuring the artery. Needle 2 enters 2 centimeters from the median line, follows the line of the vertebræ, comes in contact with the transverse process, and finally reaches the nerve, while avoiding the vertebral artery.

With a needle 9 centimeters long, a subcutaneous and subfascial band is infiltrated through the dermal wheals (Figs. 89 and 90). One hundred grams of a ½ per cent. solution of procaine-adrenin are required. This procedure may also be employed in the removal of malignant tumors.

(8) *Total Laryngectomy.*—A subcutaneous hexagon is made, extending from a point slightly above the hyoid bone to the angle of Louis.   A

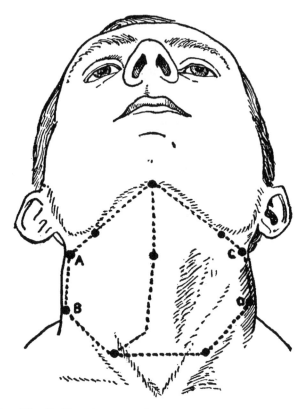

Fig. 92.—Infiltration of the anterior aspect of the neck. (*Labouré.*)   This is intended for major operations in this region, *e.g.,* for cancer of the larynx, goiter, extirpation of lymphatics of the neck for cancer of the tongue, etc.   *A, B, C,* and *D* indicate the method of paravertébral injection of the cervical nerves.   Dermal wheals are made above and below to circumscribe the operative field.

paravertebral infiltration is then conducted through two dermal wheals, as in goiter, for the purpose of anesthetizing the transverse cervical branch.

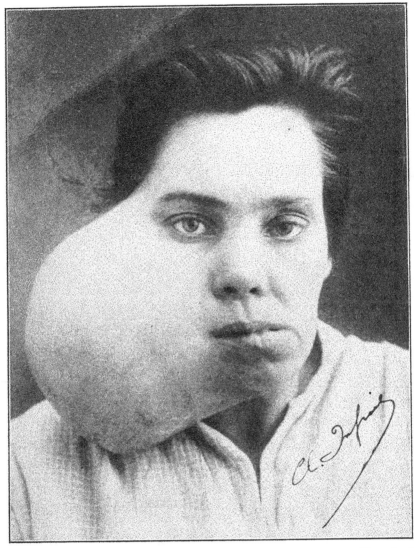

Fig. 93.—Large adamantoma of the lower maxillary. (*Pauchet.*) On the lower part of the tumor is seen a white, cross-shaped scar,— evidence of an operation carried out a few years before. This case had been recently diagnosed "inoperable sarcoma." The tumor communicated with the mouth and secreted pus abundantly. Insomnia. Liquid diet. Anesthesia was commenced by paravertebral injection of the cervical plexus, injection of the superior maxillary nerve by the orbital route, and simple infiltration of the chin and lower lip in the median line. These three anesthetizing injections enabled the operator to ligate the external carotid and perform a section from the middle of the neck to a point beyond the eyelid, extending through the chin and cheek (see the succeeding figures).

Finally, the superior laryngeal nerve is anesthetized. One must not forget to spray the pharynx

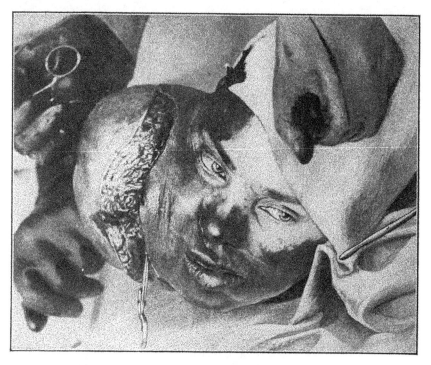

Fig. 94.—Second stage of the operation: Ligation of the
external carotid has been effected. The scalpel has just
divided the skin in front of the tumor.

with cocaine, in order to suppress the reflexes of
deglutition and prevent coughing. Two hundred
to 250 grams of a ½ per cent. solution of procaine-adrenin are required for this operation.

It is in cases such as these that regional anesthesia exhibits its superior degree of utility.

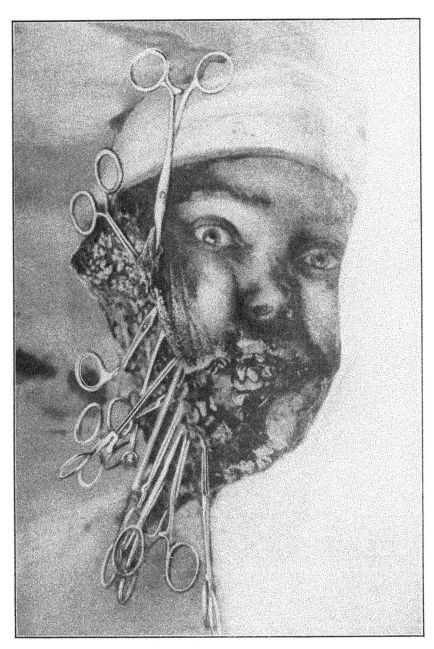

Fig. 95.—Third stage: Resection of the jaw has been completed. To the left is still seen the needle which has served to infiltrate the foramen ovale (inferior maxillary). The external carotid having been previously ligated, there is not much hemorrhage.

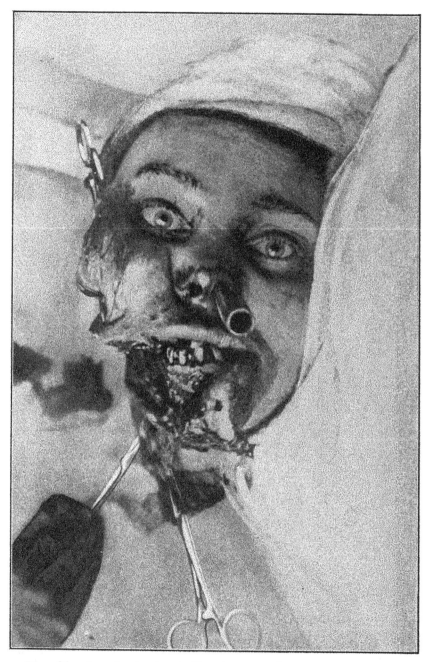

Fig. 96.—Anesthesia by infiltration of the cervical plexus and superior and inferior maxillary nerves. (*Pauchet.*) An esophageal tube has been introduced in the nose. The patient is to be fed through it.

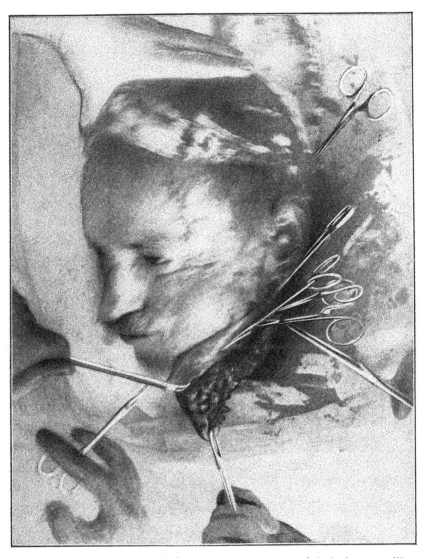

Fig. 97.—Anesthesia of the cervical plexus and inferior maxillary nerve for amputation of the tongue by the subhyoid route. (*Pauchet.*) The infrahyoid floor has been incised, and the tongue drawn out.

CHAPTER V.

ANESTHESIA OF THE THORAX AND ABDOMEN.

OPERATIONS upon the trunk may be performed under spinal anesthesia by means of cocaine (Le Filliâtre) or other drugs introduced more or less high up (Jonnesco) after a series of paravertebral injections, which constitutes the ideal regional anesthesia for the upper portions of the trunk, or by lumbosacral injections (Le Filliâtre). For intra-abdominal operations and operations in the pelvis and on the lower extremities, injection of procaine-adrenin directly into the lumbar canal offers the simplest and most complete form of anesthesia.

INTRASPINAL ANESTHESIA.

Personally we prefer regional anesthesia for all operations upon the head, face, neck and thorax, as well as all other operations of a local character. But for amputation, resection or other extensive procedures on the lower extremities, as well as for major intra-abdominal operations on the liver, stomach, intestines, and pelvic organs, intraspinal anesthesia possesses certain pronounced advantages. It is particularly valuable in operations for intestinal occlusion, as it paralyzes and softens the abdominal wall and contracts the intestine, practically eliminating the risk of fecal

(128)

vomiting and thereby aiding toward a favorable prognosis.

We do not advocate intraspinal anesthesia for any operation in which regional anesthesia is indicated, *e.g.*, in hemorrhoids, varicocele, perineorrhaphy, prostatectomy, amputation of the foot, suture of the patella, nephrectomy, cholecystotomy, and all operations on the head, neck and thorax.

The spinal cord proper terminates at about the level of the junction of the second and third lumbar vertebræ, where it becomes filiform. It is entirely safe to inject directly into the spinal canal at the space between the third and fourth (Tuffier), fourth and fifth (Chaput), and fifth lumbar vertebra and sacrum (Le Filliâtre), and, with a little care not to enter the cord, between the first and second lumbar vertebræ.

Injection into any one of the inter-vertebral spaces of the lumbar region produces insensibility of the lower part of the abdomen and the lower extremities.

Under this form of anesthesia we have performed, at the Molitor Hospital, operations upon every portion of the leg and thigh.

Some little familiarity and practice is required for the successful injection of the spinal region. It is easiest to find entrance to the canal between the last lumbar vertebra and sacrum, because here the space is wide, but as a matter of fact, it is not difficult to effect an entrance at any one of the interspaces mentioned.

Injections into the spinal canal are greatly facilitated by placing the patient in a sitting position with head bent over on the arms—the latter folded upon the knees,—and the back made to "bow" as much as possible in order to throw the spinous processes into the greatest possible prominence.

The same degree of aseptic precaution should be taken for injecting the spinal canal as for a laparotomy, both as regards the surgeon and the patient.

A strong needle of rather large caliber, 8 centimeters long, should be selected. With the index finger of the left hand the space to be injected is found, ½ centimeter from the median line of the spine, midway between two adjacent spinous processes. In the center of this space the needle is introduced in a straight line, pointing slightly inward toward the median line (Fig. 98). At a certain depth, which varies according to the conformation of the patient, the operator senses contact with the ligamenta subflava and the inter-laminar ligament, some force being required to penetrate and the operator experiencing somewhat the sensation of piercing a tense drum head. As the needle is pushed through, the silver wire is removed from its lumen from time to time to see if a drop of cerebrospinal fluid will appear. When the fluid drops more or less rapidly, according to the intraspinal tension, the syringe, containing 2 mils of a 4 per cent. solution, is adjusted, the spinal fluid slowly drawn out to complete extension of the syringe, the fluid then slowly injected in part, and the piston redrawn and reinserted several times to mix the solution with the spinal fluid and cause it to be more generally diffused

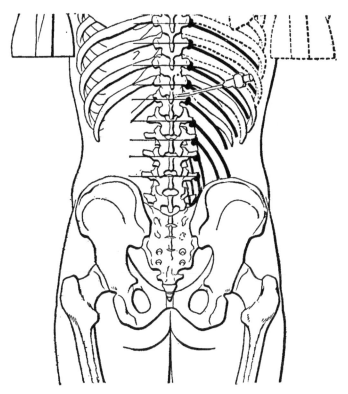

Fig. 98.—Showing point of entrance into the spinal canal. (*Pauchet.*)

in the spinal canal. When the syringe has been finally emptied into the canal, the needle is withdrawn by a quick movement, slipping the index finger of the left hand over the puncture for a moment, then touching it with a drop of iodine tincture. In from five to fifteen minutes the pa-

tient will experience complete insensibility of the
parts supplied by the nerves involved.

If the injection be made between the 12th dorsal and 1st lumbar vertebræ, it will produce a
complete anesthesia of the abdominal contents—
stomach, liver, intestines, abdominal walls—as well
as the lower extremities. If it be made between the
fifth lumbar and sacrum it will anesthetize the
perineum, anus and lower extremities. Both together are recommended for abdomino-pelvic operations such as hysterectomy or extensive extirpation of the rectum (Jonnesco).

For feeble, old individuals, and the cancerous,
cachectic, and tuberculous, it is not necessary to
employ the full strength of dose, as for the vigor-
ous patient. The anesthesia is more readily induced in the feeble.

As a precautionary measure it is well to inject, one hour before the operation, an ampoule
of scopolamine-morphine and one of strychnine or
sparteine.

Equalization of the effect of the anesthetic is
greatly facilitated by the repeated filling and partial reinjection of the contents of the syringe into
the spinal canal. If this movement is not readily
performed and something seems to prevent an
easy flow to and from the syringe, the action of
the anesthetic is likely to be imperfect.

Immediately after the injection is made the patient should be placed recumbent upon the operating table and covered warmly. For him to remain sitting up involves risk of an attack of syn-

cope. The ears should be stopped with cotton, the eyes bandaged, if necessary, and complete silence ordered. The anesthesia continues for an hour or more.

Complications.—(*a*) If cerebrospinal fluid fails to flow from the needle, either the direction of the needle is bad and the point has not penetrated the spinal canal, or the needle is plugged. Only two or three attempts are required for the operator to feel confident when he is traversing the inter-laminar ligaments separating the vertebræ. If he be satisfied that the direction of the needle is not at fault, the needle should be withdrawn, aspirated with the aid of a syringe, and reintroduced.

(*b*) If pure blood appears, the needle has penetrated a vein and must be withdrawn and reintroduced. If the liquid is mixed with blood, one should wait a moment for the fluid to become clear. To inject with bloody fluid destroys the effect of the anesthetic.

(*c*) If the liquid appears only in slow drops and will not fill the syringe ·when aspiration is made, it is useless to push the attempt farther. The needle must be withdrawn, its lumen cleared with the aid of a syringe, and the needle then reintroduced.

(*d*) Incomplete anesthesia or absence of anesthesia is due to one of the preceding errors. It does not occur in the hands of an experienced operator.

Untoward Sequelæ.—(*a*) Retention of urine

may be present for several days. The patient occasionally requires daily catheterization for a week or more.

(*b*) Vomiting after the operation is very uncommon.

(*c*) Sciatic neuralgia occurs when the operator introduces the needle to the outer side of the vertebra and pierces a nerve.

(*d*) Headache often follows the injection and lasts a week. If it is violent, lumbar puncture is necessary.

(*e*) Fecal incontinence during the operation. In the case of a total hysterectomy, this is dangerous as the fecal matter may penetrate the vagina and enter the abdominal cavity. It is wise to tampon the vagina to safeguard against this difficulty.

(*f*) Fever. The temperature may rise and fall on the first or second day; this is devoid of significance.

(*g*) Labored respiration and asphyxia have appeared where the injections have been made high up and the anesthetic has affected the center of respiration. If the mind is clear, the patient should be made to talk incessantly and draw in and blow out the air. If necessary, artificial respiration should be resorted to. As soon as the effect of the anesthetic on the medulla has passed off, natural respiration will be re-established.

(*h*) Death. Among 2000 cases Pauchet has met with 2 deaths. In 5000 cases, Jonnesco had no death. Le Filliâtre has had no deaths, either. Leyden has had 2 deaths. I consider spinal analgesia as involving the same degree of immediate danger as does chloroform.

(*i*) Nervous Manifestations. Among 5000 cases Jonnesco observed but one case of nervous disturbance. Pauchet met with one case of bladder retention which continued for three months. Organic affections not discovered by previous examination may, of course, exist, and it is certainly unjustifiable to attribute - accidents appearing a year or more after the operation to the effects of the anesthetic.

Regions Influenced.—Jonnesco has boldly praetised injection into the spinal canal along its whole length and specifies the effects of the anesthetic in the various regions as follows:—

(1) Injection between the 3d and 4th cervical vertebræ: Anesthesia of the head and neck.

(2) Cervico-dorsal injection, immediately below the vertebra prominens: Thorax and upper extremities.

(3) Between the last dorsal and first lumbar: The entire abdomen, testicles, and lower extremities.

(4) Between the last lumbar and the sacrum: The pelvis, perineum, and anus.

Injection at two points has been recommended for certain operations, viz., in operations upon the thorax, one may inject at the cervico-dorsal and dorso-lumbar levels. For abdomino-pelvic operations, one should inject at the dorso-lumbar and lumbo-sacral levels. For other operations, one injection suffices.

Pauchet says: "I do not practice injection of the spinal canal at a point above the intersection of the 12th dorsal and 1st lumbar, which insensibilizes the whole abdomen and its wall, preferring regional and local anesthesia for all operations above this level."

As in the administration of chloroform, a certain degree of danger attends the practice of spinal anesthesia, but the procedure is free of the postoperative dangers incident to general narcosis. It does not affect the viscera (lungs, liver, kidneys, or suprarenal capsules) and permits of highly traumatic operations (resection of the femur, disarticulation of the hip) with very minor evidences of shock. It renders the major abdominal operations more benign because it makes them easier, serving to contract the intestine, reducing completely the rigidity of the abdominal wall, and producing complete "abdominal silence."

There is no comparison between an operation for uterine cancer, for cancer of the rectum, and notably for acute occlusion of the intestine, under spinal anesthesia and under general narcosis.

Nerve-trunk Anesthesia.

The *thoracic nerves* emerge from the intervertebral foramina of the thoracic portion of the spine (Fig. 101). Immediately after their emergence they give an anastomotic branch to the sympathetic, and afterward divide into two branches: an *anterior* and a *posterior*. The posterior branch supplies the muscles of the back and skin in the vicinity of the midline. The anterior branches or *intercostal* nerves are situated in the intercostal spaces near the inferior borders of the ribs. They

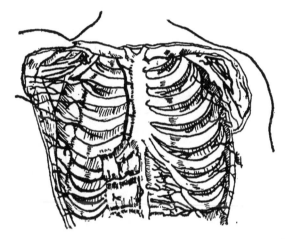

Fig. 99.—Intercostal nerves and their distribution. (*Hirschfeld.*) These nerves can be blocked by paravertebral injection or by simple intercostal injection.

are at first in contact with the pleura, near the costal angle; afterward they pass between the two intercostal muscles (Figs. 99 and 100).

The *upper dorsal nerves* (Fig. 103, D. 1, 2, and 3) supply the internal surfaces of the arm and of the forearm, and the axillary and mammary regions are supplied likewise by the succeeding nerves, down to the seventh dorsal (D. 7), inclusive. The *intercostal nerves* from the 8th to the 12th supply the thorax, and likewise the ab-

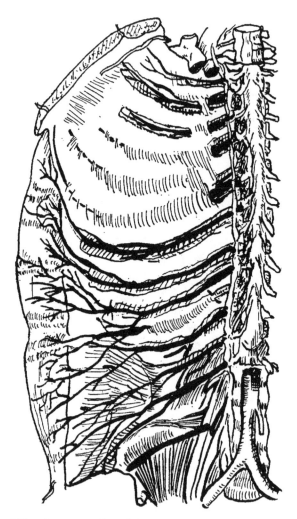

Fig. 100.—Intercostal and lumbar nerves and their distribution. (*Hirschfeld.*) The figure shows the anastomosis of these nerves with the sympathetic. The needle is introduced close enough to the vertebral column to infiltrate the communicating ramus, the viscera being thus anesthetized.

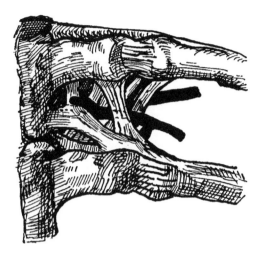

Fig. 101.—The dorsal nerves at their points of emergence. (*Testut.*) The figure shows their bifurcation into an anterior branch (intercostal) and a posterior branch which divides into two rami.

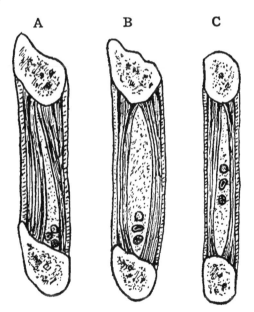

Fig. 102.—The intercostal space. (*Souligoux.*) (*A*) Posteriorly at the point of origin. (*B*) At the posterior third. (*C*) Middle portion. The internal intercostal divides to surround the blood-vessels and nerves.

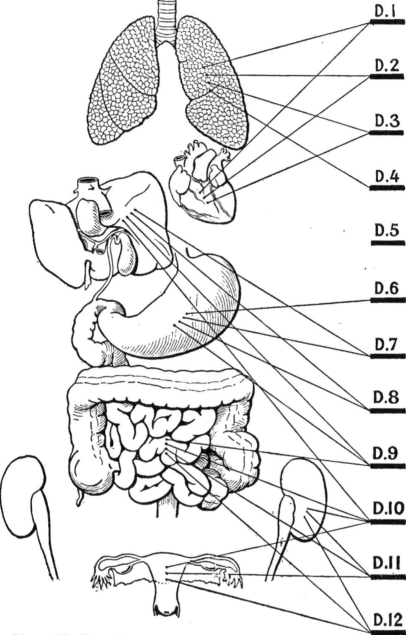

D.1
D.2
D.3
D.4
D.5
D.6
D.7
D.8
D.9
D.10
D.11
D.12

Fig. 103.—Dorsal paravertebral anesthesia for the viscera.
(*Pauchet.*) The operator is shown the dorsal points which should be
infiltrated in order to anesthetize corresponding viscera. In practice,
one should inject both higher and lower because of the anastomoses.
The lung, kidney, biliary passages, and spleen are anesthetized by an
injection made upon one side only. For other organs both sides
should be injected.

domen. Through their anastomoses with the sympathetic, they supply with sensation the following viscera: Heart (Fig. 103, D. 1, 2, and 3); lungs

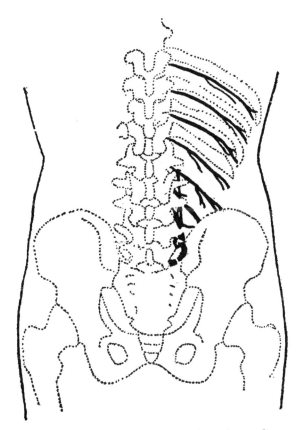

Fig. 104.—The lumbar nerves at their points of emergence. (*Pauchet.*) These nerves are accessible between the transverse processes of the lumbar vertebræ, as are the intercostals below the ribs.

(D. 1, 2, 3, and 4); stomach (D. 6, 7, 8, and 9); liver and bile ducts (D. 7, 8, 9, and 10); intestines (D. 9, 10, 11, and 12); kidneys and ureters (D. 10, 11, and 12); testicles, ovaries, and uterus

(D. 10, 11, and 12). To desensitize the viscera it is necessary to reach the anastomoses with the sympathetic (Danys).

The *lumbar nerves* are situated between the transverse processes of the lumbar vertebræ in front of the intertransverse muscles, and are surrounded by the attachments of the psoas muscle (Figs. 100, 104, 105).

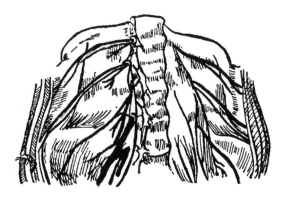

Fig. 105.—The lumbar nerves at their points of emergence. (*Hirschfeld.*)

The *ilio-hypogastric, ilio-inguinal,* and *genito-crural nerves,* supplying the anterior abdominal wall, follow, as the 12th intercostal nerves, the anterior surface of the quadratus lumborum, *i.e.,* course between this and the perirenal adipose tissue. After the 2d lumbar, the nerve trunks are so closely applied against the vertebræ that they can only be reached by injections made almost in contact with the vertebral column at a distance of 3 centimeters from the median line.

The intercostals and the 1st lumbar nerve supply not only the thoracic and abdominal wall, but also the serous membranes, the pleuræ, and the parietal peritoneum. The intermediate intercostal nerves do not anastomose at their points of origin, but from the 12th there is given off a branch to the 1st lumbar nerve. At the level of the skin the regions supplied by the respective intercostals so encroach one upon the other that the *blocking of a single nerve* does not abolish cutaneous sensation; several must be infiltrated at the upper part of the thorax to obtain complete anesthesia of a given region. The skin of the thorax also receives branches from the cervical and brachial plexuses.

The anesthesia required for operations upon the spine, thorax, and abdomen may be obtained by one of two methods.

In the case of a circumscribed operation, such as resection of one or two ribs, curettage of the sternum, operation for appendicitis, for simple hernia, etc., injections made along the course of the nerves supplying the field of operation, as described further on, will yield a complete anesthesia *limited to the parietes.* Such injections are made around, and at some distance from, the field of operation. The procedure varies for each operation in accordance with the nerve supply. This method has enabled us to dispense with general and spinal anesthesia for a number of operations, *e.g.,* in the radical cure of most voluminous hernias. It appears to us the ideal procedure for thoracotomy, and is sufficient for appendectomy when the acute attack has subsided and provided the appendix and cecum are free from adhesions. It enables us to do pylorectomy for cancer and very considerable resections of the intestines, provided the mesentery is injected in addition with a 1 per cent. solution of quinine and urea hydrochloride.

When the operation concerns unilateral viscera —kidneys, liver, spleen, bile ducts,—or any larger portion of the trunk or abdomen, it is preferable to employ the following method, which is more precise in technique and permits of covering a larger field, viz. :—

PARAVERTEBRAL ANESTHESIA.

Definition.—Paravertebral anesthesia consists in bathing the thoracic and lumbar nerves at their points of emergence from the intervertebral foramina of the dorsal and lumbar spine with a solution of procaine-adrenin. The injection anesthetizes the thoracico-abdominal wall and even the viscera through the anastomoses with the sympathetic. By injecting a 1 per cent. solution of procaine-adrenin 3 to 4 centimeters from the median line in the intervertebral spaces the surgeon is enabled to produce complete anesthesia of the thoracico-abdominal wall as well as of the unilateral viscera situated on the same side and receiving filaments of the sympathetic (liver, bile passages, spleen, kidneys, ureters).

If the operator desires to anesthetize the entire abdominal contents (intestines), two series of injections will have to be made, one to the right and the other to the left of the spinal column;

but such an event is exceptional. Paravertebral
anesthesia is useful for operations upon the thorax,

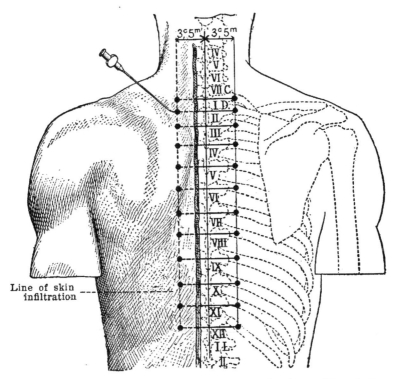

, Fig. 106.—Dorsal paravertebral anesthesia. (*Pauchet.*)
The skin is infiltrated with a band 1 centimeter wide at a distance of 35 millimeters from the median line. The operator
introduces the needle through this band and feels his way.
.The black dots show where the needle should enter to reach
the rib, somewhat laterally to the costo-vertebral articulation.
When the needle has come in contact with the rib, it turns
about its inferior border and proceeds toward a point ½ centimeter further forward and inward to reach the sympathetic
anastomosis. It should be noted that the lower angle of the
scapula corresponds to the spinous process of the seventh dorsal and the spine of the scapula to the third dorsal.

neck and abdomen, the breasts, pleuræ, lungs, and
for lateral viscera, including. the kidneys, liver,
biliary passages, pylorus, cecum, etc.

Technique.—The operator should remember that the thoracic nerves at their origin are located at equal distances from the transverse processes and at a distance of 2 centimeters in front of the intertransverse space.

The spinous processes from the first to the sixth are situated at the level of the intertransverse spaces, bounded by the two succeeding vertebræ, and at the level of the nerve immediately following. Thus, the processes D. 1 to D. 6 (Fig. 106) correspond to pairs D. 2 to D. 7. The processes D. 7 to D. 12 are situated opposite the lower portion of the corresponding intertransverse space (Fig. 110).

The lumbar nerves, at their emergence from the conjugate vertebral foramina, are situated at the level of the corresponding spinous process and slightly above the transverse process of the vertebra immediately following (Fig. 104). They are therefore accessible through the intertransverse spaces at a distance of about 3 centimeters outside the median line, and are situated *1 centimeter* in front of the transverse processes (Fig. 106 and 107).

For the Dorsal Nerves.—A needle 6 to 9 centimeters long is introduced at a point 3½ centimeters from the median line. At a depth of 4 to 5 centimeters, when the needle touches the rib, transverse process or costo-vertebral articulation, its point is inclined to reach the lower border of the bone. Then, at an angle of 25°, it is aimed at the middle line, and its progress terminated

½ a centimeter beyond. Next, 5 mils of the 1.5 per cent. solution is injected, or 7 to 8 mils of the 1 per cent. solution. It is well to move ·the

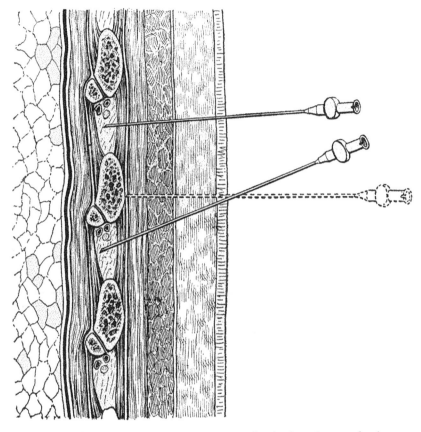

Fig. 107.—Intercostal or paravertebral dorsal anesthesia. (*Pauchet.*) The first needle is directly in the intercostal space and in the vicinity of the nerve. The second (dotted line) has at first come in contact with the rib, but has then been given an oblique direction downward and has reached the vicinity of the nerve.

point of the needle to and fro in order to be sure that the nerve is well bathed and to include the anastomosis of the sympathetic and the posterior

as well as the anterior branch of the spinal root
(Fig. 108).

Two difficulties may arise:

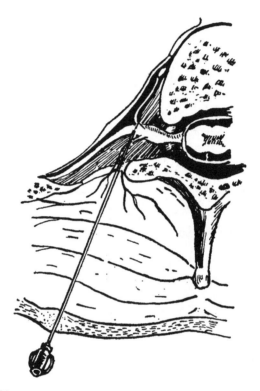

Fig. 108.—Paravertebral dorsal anesthesia. (*Pauchet* and
Sourdat.)   The needle enters at a point 35 millimeters from
the median line, close to the inferior border of the rib; then,
at a point 1 centimeter anterior and internal, it reaches the
nerve root and impregnates the anastomosis with the sympathetic.

(*a*) *If blood comes from the needle,* a vein
has been wounded.   The position of the needle
must be changed, otherwise the injection will pass
into the vein, and no anesthesia will be produced.
It is important to bear in mind that when this

accident happens, the patient turns pale and experiences nausea.

(*b*) *Penetration into the pleura* will cause

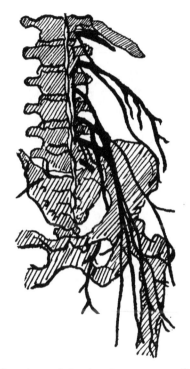

Fig. 109.—Direction of the lumbar nerves after their emergence from the conjugate foramina. (*Pauchet.*) To reach these nerves, the needle is inserted at a distance of 3 centimeters outside of the spinous process. In the case of the intercostals, at a distance of 3½ centimeters, with the needle close to the lower border of the rib, one reaches the nerve numbered one less than the spinous process serving as landmark. In the case of the lumbar nerves, the needle, introduced at the level of the spinous process, will pass above the upper border of the corresponding transverse process and come in contact with the nerve of the same number.

the patient to cough. The needle should be withdrawn and inclined slightly outward. This accident, likewise, presents the disadvantage that the

anesthetic is absorbed without producing anesthesia. To obviate it, one should avoid introducing
the needle more than 1 centimeter after having

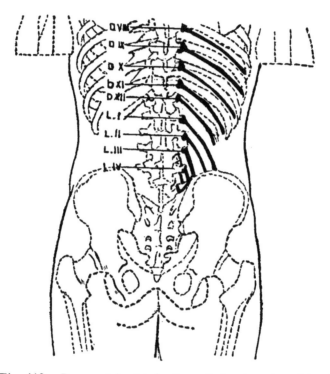

Fig. 110.—Paravertebral injection of the dorsal and lumbar
region. (*Pauchet*.) The needle enters at a point 3½ centimeters outside of the dorsal spinous process. Reaching the
lower border of the rib, it then inclines slightly inward, ad-
vances 1 centimeter, and attains the anastomosis of the sympathetic, thus anesthetizing the viscera.

passed the transverse process, or at a distance of
½ centimeter below the rib itself.

For the Lumbar Nerves.—The needle is introduced at a distance of 3 centimeters from the
median line. After the transverse process has
been found, at a depth of 4 to 5 centimeters, the

superior border is followed around, the point pushed in for another centimeter, and the injection made (Figs. 109 and 110).

Dermal infiltration is employed at first, and a straight -band, corresponding to the roots to be injected and parallel with the median line, traced on the surface of the skin. The band referred to should be traced as follows:

A very fine, sharp-pointed needle 3 to 5 centimeters in length is used. The skin is marked with a dermal pencil at a distance of 3½ centimeters from the median line (it is difficult to follow this line exactly without deviation if there is no landmark). A strip of skin 1 centimeter wide is now infiltrated with the patient sitting bowed forward and the shoulders well drawn in as for spinal anesthesia, or lying down on his side.

This having been accomplished, the operator, employing a needle 6 or 9 centimeters long—according to its strength—begins injecting the nerves. The introduction of the needle will be painless. Each spinous process is sought with the left index finger (a difficult matter in stout people), and at the level of the spinous process the needle is introduced 3½ centimeters from the median line until it meets the rib or transverse process. In muscular subjects the inexperienced operator must feel his way. When the point strikes the rib, it should be withdrawn, then directed against and past the lower costal border until the bony resistance disappears. The operator now continues to push the needle ½ centimeter beyond and injects 5 to 8 mils of the 1 per cent. solution, at the same time executing a to and fro movement in order not to miss bathing the nerve. The injection having been completed, *the needle is allowed to remain in place* to serve as a landmark. The operator then locates the spinous process of the next vertebra below, and at its level and exactly below the needle above, he introduces his second needle and begins as before. For the third injection, the second needle is left in place as a landmark and, if necessary, the first needle used for the injection.

After the injections are finished about fifteen minutes are required for the anesthesia to take full effect. The intercostal space, muscles, pleura, sternum, and ribs are all rendered insensible. The skin anesthesia begins one or two interspaces below the first injection. Transversely, it occupies the intercostal space; anteriorly it reaches the median line, and posteriorly, it often stops behind the point where the injections have been made. If the injections have been practised at points immediately external to the conjugate foramen, the posterior branch is also blocked and a *laminectomy* can be effected.

Sixty to 80 grams of the 1 per cent. solution suffice for the anesthetization of 12 nerves. An absolute anesthesia of the thoracic wall is thus obtained which extends both anteriorly and posteriorly to the midline.

For the upper portion of the thorax, the functions of the cervical plexus must be also interrupted. A subcutaneous band· must be infiltrated the length of the clavicle and spine of the scapula. If the field of operation involves the axilla or the supraclavicular fossa, the brachial plexus should be anesthetized.

For thoracic operations involving only the ribs and parietes, there is no objection to substituting intercostal anesthesia for the paravertebral anesthesia, *i.e.,* instituting the anesthesia at a more lateral point on the course of the intercostal nerve above the region to be operated upon. The technique of this procedure will be described later.

PARACENTESIS OF THE PLEURAL CAVITY.

With a 3-centimeter needle, the course to· be followed by the trocar passing in from the skin to the pleura is injected. A ½ per cent. solution proves sufficient; such anesthesia permits of the use of large trocars without pain.

THORACOTOMY FOR EMPYEMA WITH COSTAL RESECTION.

The operator is given the choice between a paravertebral anesthesia or the less radical intercostal or pericostal anesthesia, the technique of which is as follows:

. Attention is directed to Fig. 111, which represents three adjacent ribs. Upon the middle one, the part in black is to be resected; there will therefore be two intercostal spaces to anesthetize. Four wheals are marked out and through these 5 mils of the 1 per cent. solution injected into the thickness of the intercostal muscles. The needle point seeks the upper rib and follows its inferior border until it passes beyond.

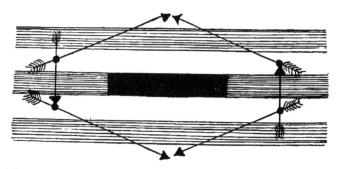

Fig. 111.—Resection of a rib. (*Sourdat.*) An injection is made in the adjacent intercostal spaces forward and backward on the portion of rib to be resected, and followed by peripheral infiltration, subcutaneously and intramuscularly.

The muscles and subcutaneous tissue are infiltrated with 30 or 40 mils of the ½ per cent. solution in the direction of the arrows. The resulting anesthesia is complete; yet it is well to bear in mind that the patient will complain if any traction is made on the ribs, producing torsion of the costo-vertebral ligaments. The patient may also complain if he hears the section of the ribs: it is therefore well to cut the ribs gently and to stop the patient's ears. A little girl 11 years of age—the niece of a colleague,—upon whom we did a resection of 3 ribs for interlobar empyema,

· cried every time she heard the cutting of a rib, though she had not complained once during the remainder of the operation, except during the production of the dermal wheals. A man 30 years of age cried out when he heard a costal cartilage fall into the bucket on the floor.

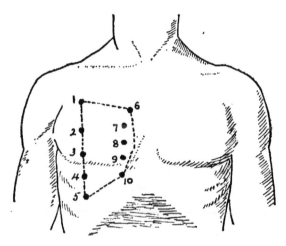

Fig. 112.—Resection of the costal cartilages. Diagram of the infiltration for mobilization of the ribs, as for emphysema. The zone of anesthesia should be extended downward to the free border of the ribs if it is desired to remove a section of cartilage to be used for filling in a bony gap in the skull from trephining.

RESECTION OF THE SECOND TO THE FIFTH COSTAL
CARTILAGES FOR RIGIDITY OF THE THORAX.

From the 2d to the 5th interspace two rows of wheals are made (Fig. 112)—the outer at the external ends of the cartilages, the inner along the sternum. Through each point 5 mils of the

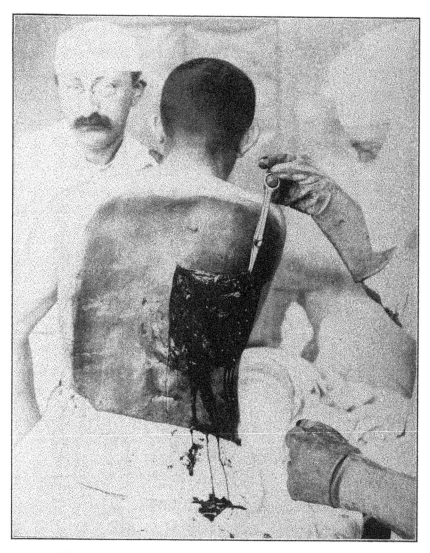

Fig. 113.—Extensive pleurotomy and costal resection for pleural sinus. Raising the flap of soft tissues.

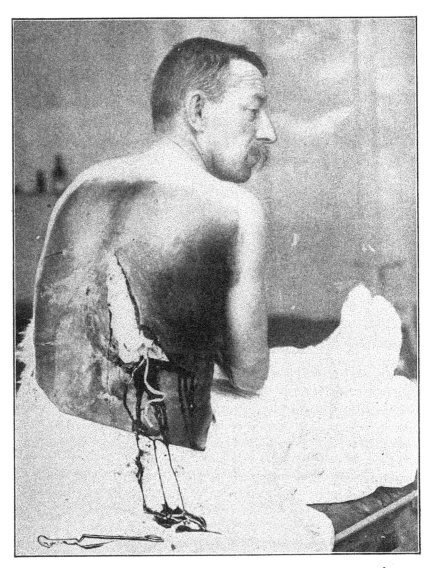

Fig. 114.—Extensive pleurotomy and costal resection for pleural sinus. (*Pauchet.*) The wound tamponed at the close of the operation.

1 per cent. solution are injected to enclose the
field of operation in the dotted line, finishing with
50 mils of the ½ per. cent. solution. The same
procedure is followed for operations involving the
pericardium and heart, or for subphrenic abscess
or suppurative costo-chondritis. When decortication of the lung is practised for a pleural sinus,
it should be remembered that in patients who
have undergone costal resections the ribs have become welded together. Under these conditions it
is indispensable to employ paravertebral anesthesia, intercostal infiltration being no longer possible.

OPERATIONS UPON THE STERNUM.

Five mils. of the 1 per cent. solution are injected on both sides in each space close to the
sternum. The skin and subcutaneous tissues at a
distance are then infiltrated with the ½ per cent.
solution of procaine-adrenin.

THORACOTOMY FOR ABSCESS OF THE LUNG, EX-
TRACTION OF FOREIGN BODIES, OPENING OF
INTERLOBAR ABSCESS, REMOVAL OF
TUMOR OF THE LUNGS, ETC.

A very wide anesthesia of the intercostal nerves
at their origin should be instituted. The operator
may either employ paravertebral anesthesia or infiltrate the intercostal nerves at points 5 centimeters outside of the line of the spinous proc-

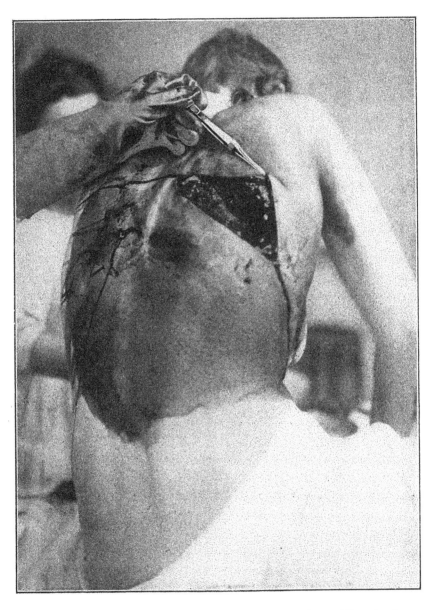

Fig. 115.—Wound made for resection of two ribs. (*Pauchet.*)
Interlobar pleurisy.

esses, *i.e.*, at the lateral border of the mass of the spinal muscles. The intercostal spaces are more easily found in this situation than elsewhere.

The operator traces a line with a dermal pencil at a distance of 5 centimeters from the spinous processes. Then, with a very fine and sharp needle 6 centimeters long, a band 1 centimeter wide is infiltrated with the ½ per cent. solution along this line, with the patient sitting down, bent forward, and with the shoulders drawn inward; or lying down on the side. Along this line and on a level with each spinous process, an injection is made immediately below the corresponding rib. Paravertebral anesthesia, which renders the lung insensitive, is the procedure of choice.

Operations for Tumor of the Breast.

For benign operations on the breast, including extirpation of adenoma and total extirpation of the mammary gland, a large subcutaneous lozenge, is circumscribed through 4 or 5 wheals. Next, the submammary tissue is infiltrated, thus completing an absolute circumferential anesthesia. A large amount of ½ per cent. solution—100 or 150 mils—is required. Half of the liquid runs off with the blood during the operation. We have injected as much as 250 mils without any harmful after-effects.

REMOVAL OF CANCER OF THE BREAST.

Procaine-adrenin has been used by us several times for this purpose, not only in thin women, but also in fat women with some contraindication to general anesthesia, such as renal insufficiency, myocarditis, etc. The results were good. At times inhalation of ethyl chloride became necessary, however, at the time of dissection of the axilla.

The technique comprises the following steps: (*a*) Blocking of the brachial plexus with 10 mils of the 1 per cent. solution, injected from above the clavicle or in the axilla. The latter route presents the added advantage of anesthetizing simultaneously the surrounding cellular tissues. (*b*) Paravertebral injection from D. 1 to D. 10 with 50 mils of 1 per cent. solution. (*c*) Subcutaneous injection of 100 mils of ½ per cent. procaine-adrenin, starting at the acromion, following the clavicle to block the cervical plexus, then the midline of the thorax, the lower border of the thorax, and finally passing backward to the prominence of the latissimus dorsi. In the case of an obese woman, we employ ordinarily 150 mils of procaine-adrenin; large amounts of the fluid run off, however, during the operation. By the use of hypotonic saline solution the dose of procaine-adrenin injected may be reduced.

Operations in the Axilla.

Theoretically, the brachial plexus may be blocked by supraclavicular injection and the first 5 intercostal nerves by paravertebral injection. To the inexperienced operator we advise, however, merely an infiltration of the axilla, as explained later.

ABDOMEN.

If the operative procedure required consists merely of incising an anterior peritoneal abscess. appendicular or otherwise, simple infiltration of the wall by Reclus's method is sufficient. For an operation involving prolonged maneuvers, such as exploration of the abdomen, recourse must be had to anesthesia of the wall at a distance and to paravertebral anesthesia.

(*A*) *Infiltration of the wall at a distance* from the field of operation results in a block of the nerve supply and yields a perfect anesthesia, but one which is only parietal. While the viscera are not reached, the incision, separation, and suture of the abdominal wall are rendered painless. The viscera, furthermore, are only slightly sensitive provided *no traction* be exerted. This semi-sensibility on their part permits of the performance of gastro-enterostomies and intestinal resections under parietal infiltration, without shock.

In some instances, after the abdomen has been opened, the anesthesia can be continued by direct injection of *quinine and urea solution* into the mesentery. One mil of a 1 per cent. solution may be injected into the meso-appendix for appendicectomy, and a few drops of a 1 per cent. solution in the vicinity of each omental vessel for resection of the omentum. Such injections between the two layers of the peritoneum, along the vessels, gives a perfect anesthesia; but it is only practicable in certain special cases. For resection of the stomach, for instance, we anesthetize the nerves of the organ by infiltrating the peritoneum in the vicinity of the coronary artery, the pylorus, and the two gastric omenta. Only very gentle handling is, however, permissible, or during painful manipulations some drops of ethyl chloride, chloroform, or ether will have to be administered. The anesthesia is often incomplete, demanding either some mental encouragement of the patient or a few whiffs of an anesthetic. In three-fourths of the cases this method proves effective, and permits of the performance of severe operations without shock.

(*B*) *Paravertebral anesthesia,* on the other hand, gives absolute anesthesia, at least on the side of the body on which it is made. It must be bilateral if the viscera are in or pass beyond the median line. A choledochotomy, or removal of a tumor of the cecum, can be perfectly performed under right-sided paravertebral anesthesia. For a nephrectomy, or the removal of a circumscribed tumor of the colon, unilateral anesthesia is likewise sufficient. To operate on the stomach (gastrectomy) or pancreas, however, both sides must be injected.

The operator may manipulate throughout the abdomen by infiltrating from the 5th intercostal to the 2d lumbar nerve on both sides. The required 22 injections are, however, distressing and involve the use of a large dose of procaine-adrenin.

On several occasions we have made a transverse bilateral incision after paravertebral infiltration of only 6 nerves on each side; the anesthesia was perfect. For the stomach, we do not employ this procedure systematically because we prefer the long vertical incision, and we confine the anesthesia to simple infiltration of the abdominal wall with injection of quinine and urea in the mesentery. The two forms of anesthesia may be combined by (a) making a double paravertebral injection of the D. 6, 7, 8, and 9 nerves,—8 injections all told, 4 on each side—to anesthetize the stomach and epigastric wall, and (b) infiltrating in the midline below the umbilicus for a distance of 5 to 6 centimeters with a weak anesthetic solution.

Practice with paravertebral injections induces the surgeon to employ them more and more frequently in his work, as they are particularly adapted for abdominal surgery. The more experienced the surgeon in the technique, the more inclined he becomes to substitute the procedure for parietal infiltration. I shall present, however, with reference to each operation, the details of the latter, pointing out at the same time the precautions to be taken during the course of the operation under regional anesthesia.

OPERATIONS UPON THE STOMACH.

GASTROSTOMY AND GASTRO-ENTEROSTOMY.

Three dermal wheals are infiltrated,—one at the level of the ensiform cartilage, the others at

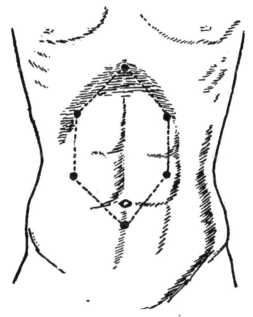

Fig. 116.—Infiltration for supraumbilical laparotomy. Six wheals. For gastrectomy and gastroenterostomy.

the free borders of the ribs 10 or 12 centimeters from the first. The subcutaneous cellular tissues and portions of muscle attached to the costal border are infiltrated successively in order to block the nerve filaments that supply the midline over two-thirds of its length above the umbilicus. The abdominal wall can then be immediately incised, either to the right or left of this line. Next, the skin and muscles over the free borders of the ribs on the left side are infiltrated for a distance of 10, 12, or 15 centimeters.

Manipulations of the stomach being but slightly painful, all complementary anesthesia is useless. The infiltration requires from 100 to 120 mils of the weak solution to completely relax the abdominal muscles. Such anesthesia is sufficient also for gastro-enterostomy. We inject previously, however, pantopon or scopolamine-morphine.

GASTRECTOMY.

The same paracostal incision is made, but in a bilateral form (Fig. 117). The operation is rather more painful owing to the extensive and prolonged manipulation of the stomach involved. If a complete anesthesia is considered advisable, it is necessary either to institute a double paravertebral anesthesia (6 nerves on each side) or after the abdomen is opened to give some whiffs of chloroform or infiltrate the mesentery with quinine and urea. It will be sufficient to chloroform the patient slightly during the liberation and exploration. The suturing and cutting of the intestines are painless. The mental condition of the patient is all-important. There are great contrasts between individual temperaments. Some patients do not utter a word during the operation, while others cry out for an anesthetic and never cease complaining.

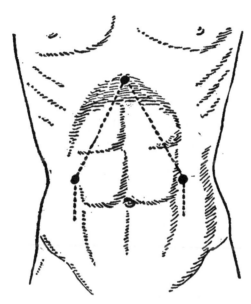

Fig. 117.—Infiltration for high laparotomy. (*Sourdat.*) Yields a larger area of anesthesia than the preceding. For gastro-enterostomy; operations on the gall-bladder and colon.

MEDIAN HYPOGASTRIC INCISION.

We seldom practice abdomino-pelvic operations under local anesthesia. Yet the evacuation of a tuberculous ascites or the removal of a movable tumor of the ovary may be very easily effected with this procedure. The pedicle should be infiltrated with a 1 per cent. solution of quinine and

urea without injecting the viscera; it can then
be easily crushed and tied without pain.

Cesarean section can readily be practised under
infiltration anesthesia. A lozenge-shaped area
three finger-breadths wide, in the median line, is
infiltrated so as to block the musculo-cutaneous
endings of the abdominal nerves. Opening of the
abdomen is thus rendered painless, the peritoneum
having been anesthetized by the blocking of the
parietal nerves. The uterus is almost insensitive;
yet it is well to anesthetize it with quinine and
urea, infiltrating a strip of uterine tissue on each
side of the intended uterine section at a distance
of two or three finger-breadths from the median
line. There is little bleeding.

In *hysterectomy,* as for cancer, fibroids, or sal-
pingitis, we prefer lumbar spinal anesthesia, but
bilateral paravertebral anesthesia will also serve
the purpose. One must inject twelve pairs on
each side,—the six lower intercostals, three lumbar, and three sacral. For the lesser operations,
such as hysteropexy, removal of ovarian cysts,
etc., we prefer a brief general anesthesia.

Hypogastric anesthesia for cystotomy is instituted through two wheals, the one at the umbilicus and the other at the pubis. Through these
one infiltrates, not in the median line, but on
either side, the skin and muscles. The peritoneum
is itself anesthetized. The muscles must be anesthetized, and not the linea alba,—that they may be
separated without pain.

OPERATIONS IN THE ILIAC FOSSA.
ILEOCECAL REGION.

Here it is well to institute a sufficiently low paravertebral anesthesia, *i.e.,* one involving the last two intercostal nerves and the first three lumbar. If, owing to the technical difficulties, the operator prefers to block the nerves nearer the

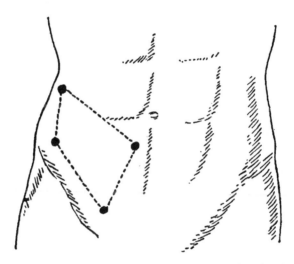

Fig. 118.—Infiltration for operative work in the ileocecal region. (*Pauchet.*) A diamond-shaped figure under the skin and in the muscles, circumscribing the future incision, should be infiltrated. For appendicitis; ileocecal resection.

field of operation, he can have recourse to infiltration of the abdominal wall in the following manner (see Fig. 118 and the subsequent illustrations).

Four dermal wheals are made, in the form of a lozenge. The two lateral wheals are placed, the one inside the anterior superior spine of the ilium, the other, two or three finger-breadths from

the middle line. The superior and inferior wheals
are situated, the one at a distance of three finger-
breadths from the first, the other, three finger-
breadths from the second. The muscular layers
should be infiltrated only at the two upper sides
of the lozenge; over the two lower sides only the

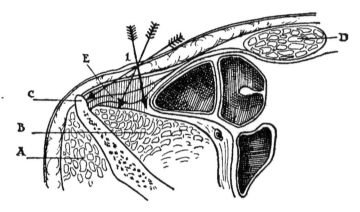

Fig. 119.—Deep "fan-shaped" injection to infiltrate the muscular mass at the point of emergence of the nerves of the inguino-crural region. (*Pauchet.*) (*D*) Rectus abdominis. (*B*)
Ilio-psoas. (*A*) Gluteus. (C) Iliac bone. (*E*) Three directions of the needle: the first perpendicular to the skin, toward
the subserous cellular tissue; the second, parallel to the skin,
beneath the aponeurosis; the third, intermediate, oblique in the
intermuscular space, where the nerves are found. (1) Dermal
wheal.

subcutaneous cellular tissue is to be infiltrated.
The infiltration of the muscles produces not only
anesthesia of these structures, but also anesthesia
of the peritoneum.

With this procedure we have performed the
following operations: Cecostomy, resection of the
ileocecal segment for cancer or tuberculosis, appendicectomy, closing of intestinal fistula, and en-
terostomy.

The incision in the abdominal wall and the separation of the wound margins are painless, but it is necessary to infiltrate the meso-appendix or the end of the mesentery with quinine and urea if section - of this last structure is indicated.

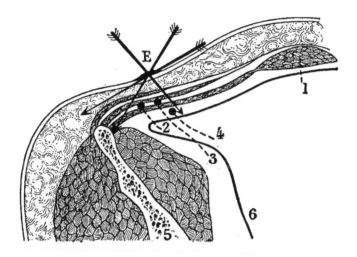

Fig. 120.—Same as the preceding. (*Pauchet.*) Horizontal section at the level of the iliac spine. (1) Rectus abdominis. (2) and (3) Ilio-hypogastric and ilio-inguinal nerves, situated at this point between the internal oblique and transversalis muscles. (4) Genito-crural nerve. (5) Iliac bone. (6) Parietal peritoneum. (*E*) Wheal situated two finger-breadths within the iliac spine and through which the fan-shaped injection is made.

On the whole, I desire to emphasize the fact that paravertebral anesthesia for the viscera is rather to be recommended. The operation for appendicitis may almost always be performed under it. We have operated upon children of 8 years, and with greater facility children of 10 to 15 years, without general anesthesia.

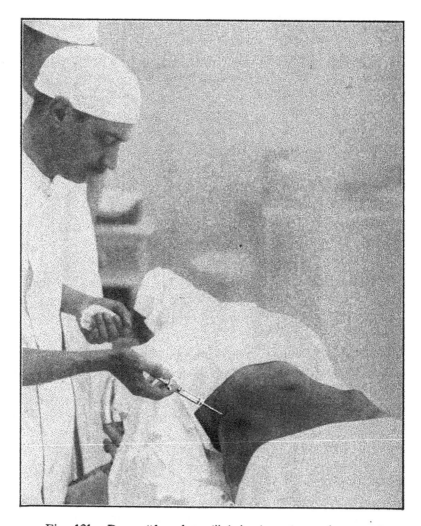

Fig. 121.—Deep, "fan-shaped" injection above the anterior superior iliac spine. (*Pauchet* and *Sourdat.*) To anesthetize the wall of the iliac fossa, for appendectomy, cecostomy, ileocecal resection. The figure shows the manner of direct injection, perpendicular to the plane of the wall.

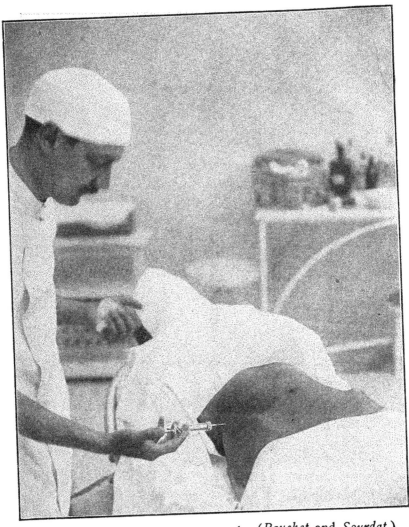

Fig. 122.—Oblique injection upward. (*Pauchet* and *Sourdat.*)
Note the direction imparted to the syringe and needle.

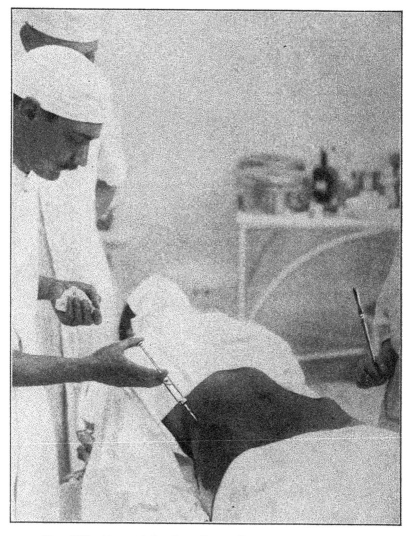

Fig. 123.—Same injection directed obliquely downward.
(*Pauchet* and *Sourdat.*)

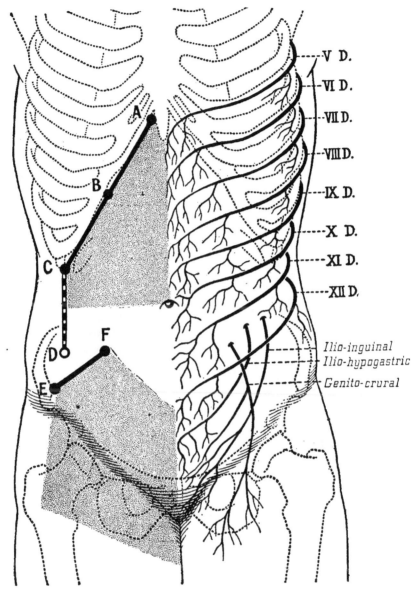

Fig. 124.—Paracostal anesthesia—costo-iliac and para-iliac. (*Pauchet.*) Anesthesia of the entire abdominal wall (anesthetized zone in gray). To the right are seen the intercostal filaments supplying the abdominal wall, and lower down the ilio-hypogastric and ilio-inguinal nerves, and the genito-crural (vertically directed). To the left of the figure, *A, B,* and C show the paracostal infiltration of a portion of muscle and of the skin (stomach, liver, and duodenum). *C, D,* anesthesia of the abdominal wall for the ascending colon. *E. F.* useful for cecal or appendicular operations and for the radical cure of inguinal hernia.

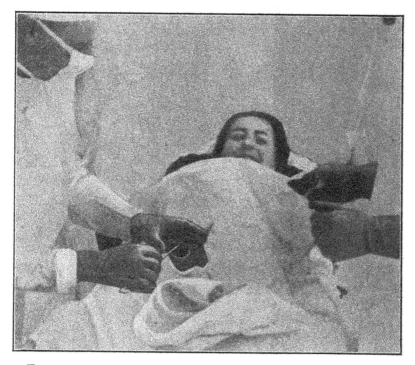

Fig. 125.—Appendicitis. (*Pauchet* and *Sourdat*.) Incision of the abdominal wall.

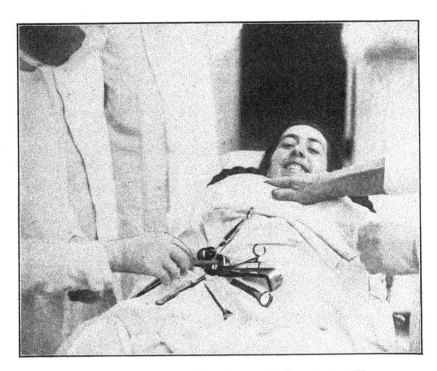

Fig. 126.—Appendicitis. (*Pauchet* and *Sourdat.*) The appendix and cecum are brought to the exterior.

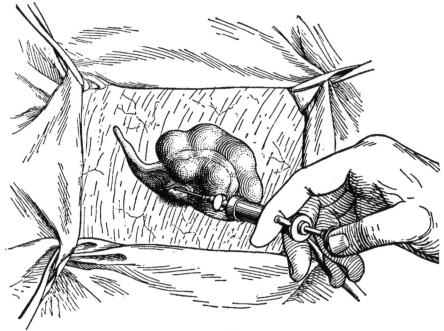

Fig. 127.—Anesthesia of the meso-appendix. (*Pauchet.*)
Interval operation. The needle is inserted between the two
layers of the meso-appendix, in the vicinity of the appendicular
artery. One mil of ½ per cent. quinine and urea hydrochloride
solution is injected. The operator may then tie and divide,
without pain, the meso-appendix and the appendix itself.

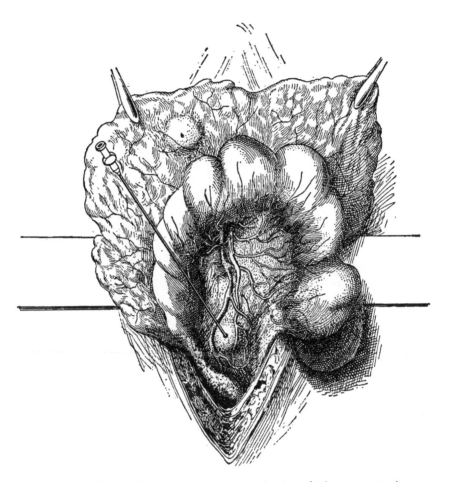

Fig. 128.—Quinine and urea anesthesia of the mesenteric nerves before intestinal resection. (*Pauchet.*) The needle is inserted in the first layer of the mesentery, and 1 or 2½ mils of ½ per cent. quinine and urea solution injected. The operator is enabled immediately to cut the vascular pedicle and resect the intestine without pain. In this instance, it is the transverse colon.

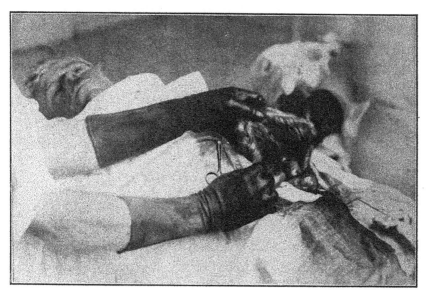

Fig. 129.—Pylorectomy for callous ulcer. (*Pauchet.*) First step: Exploration of the abdomen. (Patient from the La Pitié Hospital).

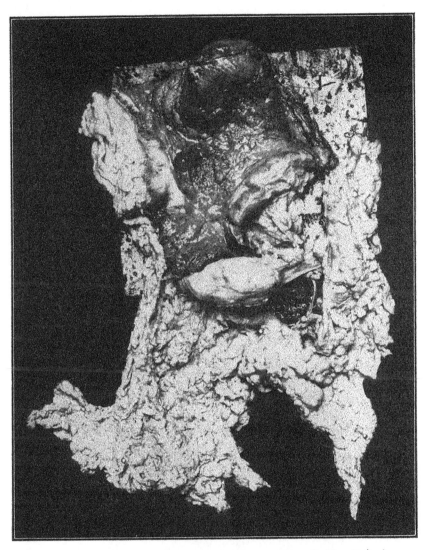

Fig. 130.—Pylorectomy for callous ulcer. (*Pauchet.*) Pyloric segment resected. The canal has been incised lengthwise along the greater curvature, then spread out. Lower down, the great omentum is seen attached to the greater curvature by an inflamed lymph-gland. The operative mortality is 8 per cent.

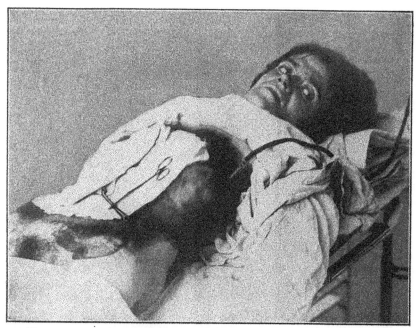

Fig. 131.—Continent jejunostomy. (*Pauchet.*) For a large
cancer of the stomach. (Patient from La Pitié Hospital).

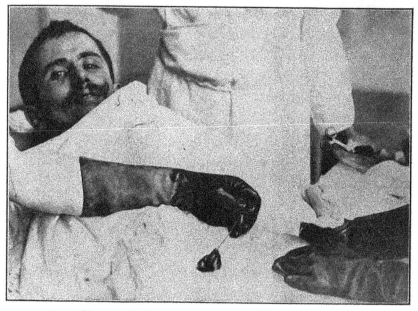

Fig. 132.—Artificial anus due to wound of the intestine.
(*Pauchet.*) Military wound from La Pitié Hospital (shell
splinter). Circular enterorrhaphy.

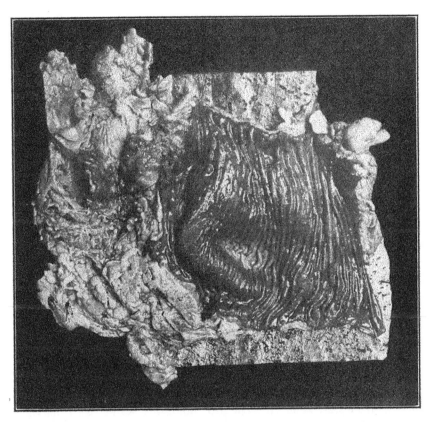

Fig. 133.—Ileocecal segment invaded by cicatricial tuberculosis. (*Pauchet.*) To the right the end of the small intestine may be recognized. The cecum has become transformed into a fibrous mass, with a small, hardly perceptible, mucous canal. (La Pitié Hospital.)

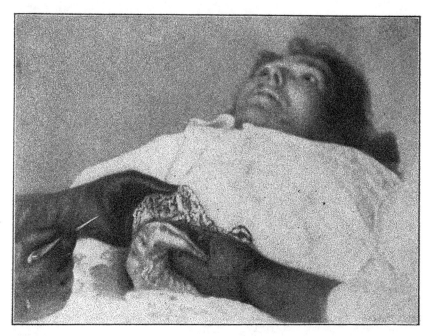

Fig. 134.—Partial gastrectomy for saddle ulcer of the lesser curvature. (*Pauchet.*)   First stage of the operation: Separation of the omentum by means of the scalpel.   The assistant holds the transverse colon with the left hand; the operator holds the scalpel with his right hand and with the left the omentum is separated from the transverse colon for examination of the posterior surface of the stomach.   Mortality 8 per cent.

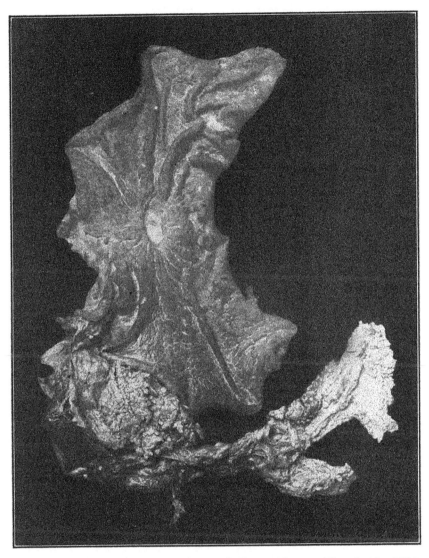

Fig. 135.—Specimen from the preceding patient. (*Pauchet.*) Middle segment of the stomach, showing a saddle ulcer of the lesser curvature. The resected segment has been laid open along the greater curvature, to which the omentum is attached below. The center of the figure, where the ulcer is found, corresponds to the middle of the lesser curvature.

Umbilical Hernia.

Umbilical hernias and hernias of the linea alba are operated under lateral infiltration of the muscles, in the same manner as for laparotomy. The operator infiltrates successively the skin and the

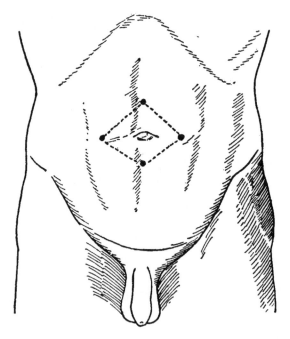

Fig. 136.—Anesthesia for radical cure of a reducible umbilical hernia. (*Pauchet.*) Through the wheals a ring of infiltration is made, following the dotted line, under the skin and in the thickness of the muscles.

muscles down to the subserous cellular tissue with a weak solution. Pauchet, in 1914, operated at Amiens on an obese woman with a strangulated hernia in the median line, of the size of an adult's head and containing 1.50 meters of gangrenous intestine. The patient complained somewhat when

the mesentery was ligated, but it did not become
necessary to have her inhale any chloroform. Two
hundred and fifty mils of a ½ per cent. solution
were employed.

In an extremely obese woman with a simple
umbilical hernia, Pauchet injected as much as 300

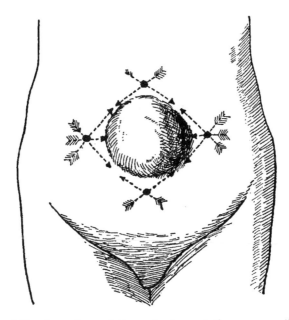

Fig. 137.—Location of the wheals and the proper direction
of injection for anesthetization in irreducible umbilical hernia.
(*Pauchet.*)

mils of the weak solution. Part of the fluid es-
caped, however, during the operation. In making
these injections, 12-centimeter needles were employed.

For all these operations, the procedure is always the same. A lozenge-shaped wall of infiltration around the umbilicus is established. Through
four wheals all of the subcutaneous ; tissue and

muscles are infiltrated, following the lines that form the lozenge. In cases of umbilical hernia and post-operative eventration, injection of quinine and urea into the omentum, about the vessels, is

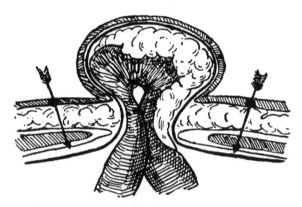

Fig. 138.—Injection for irreducible umbilical hernia. (*Pauchet.*) The infiltration is conducted at a distance from the ring and through the entire thickness of the wall.

an important preliminary to resection of the omental membrane, which under this treatment becomes absolutely insensitive.

Inguinal Hernia.

The operation for inguinal hernia is without doubt, of all operations, that in which regional anesthesia gives the greatest satisfaction, no matter how voluminous the hernia may be. That it is indicated is due to three factors: (1) The disease itself is hardly more dangerous than general anesthesia; the latter may give rise to a bronchitis that is prejudicial to consolidation at the points of suture; (2) the resultant vomiting has the same tendency; (3) regional anesthesia, which, it must be recognized, is imperfect for certain operations, shows its utility for the radical cure

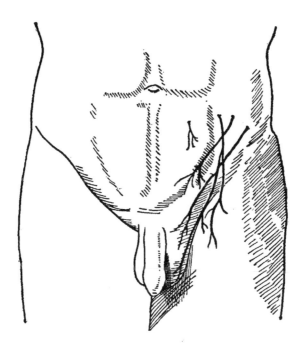

Fig. 139.—Nerve supply of the inguinal region (diagrammatic). (*Pauchet.*) Points of emergence of the genito-crural, ilio-hypogastric, ilio-inguinal, and of an anterior branch of the 12th intercostal. For anesthesia of the inguino-crural region they should be reached here by injection. The needle should be introduced within the anterior superior iliac spine.

of inguinal hernia when properly employed, and the technique for this operation is very simple. In April, 1916, at the La Pitié Hospital we operated on an inguinal hernia of the size of a large adult's head, without the slightest pain.

Paravertebral anesthesia will yield a perfect anesthesia at a distance and seems to us the procedure of election. No matter how large the hernia, it will be sufficient to inject the two lower intercostal and upper three or four lumbar nerves. Yet the great majority of surgeons prefer anesthesia by localized infiltration of the nerves of the region, the technique of which is as follows:

Figures 139 and 124 show the innervation of the groin and of the crural region respectively. The genital branch of the genito-crural reaches the spermatic cord through the internal ring and accompanies it in the canal and in the skin of the scrotum or of the labia majora. The ilio-inguinal is situated above the iliac spine, between the oblique muscles; it passes under the aponeurosis of the external oblique, emerges from the inguinal canal upon the anterior surface of the cord and of the sac, and ends in the skin of the scrotum or mons veneris. The ilio-hypogastric, parallel to the preceding and slightly higher up, makes its way between the two oblique muscles; reaching the inguinal region, it passes under the aponeurosis of the external oblique, crosses through the anterior layer of the sheath of the rectus, and ends in the skin of the groin. These three nerves anastomose with each other. It is necessary, therefore, that all three be anesthetized. They are all to be found grouped together in a space of 2 or 3 finger-breadths within and above the iliac spine.

REDUCIBLE INGUINAL HERNIA.

Two wheals are made, the first two finger-breadths within the anterior superior iliac spine and the second corresponding to the pubis at the

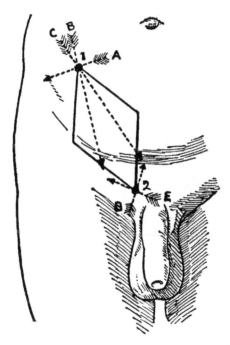

Fig. 140.—Anesthesia for irreducible inguinal hernia. (*Sourdat.*) Location of the two wheals. The arrows show the direction of the deep injections. The unbroken line outlines the subcutaneous infiltration.

level of the external abdominal ring. Through wheal No. 1, infiltration is executed according to the scheme shown by the arrows in Figs. 119 and 120. All the muscular layers situated between point 1 and the ilium are infiltrated, using

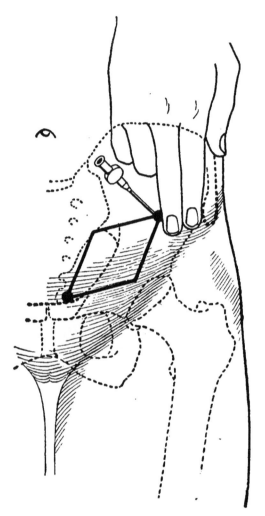

Fig. 141.—Same as the preceding. (*Sourdat.*) A wheal is made two finger-breadths within the anterior superior iliac spine. The second wheal is made above the horizontal ramus of the pubis. The black line shows the subcutaneous infiltration.

20 mils of a 1 per cent. solution. A 9-centimeter needle is introduced perpendicularly, passing through the aponeurosis of the external oblique, the internal oblique, and the transversalis muscle. It is then inserted so as to cover a fan-shaped sector, and more and more obliquely toward the spine of the ilium. The muscular layer here is very thick. This injection reaches the ilio-hypogastric and ilio-inguinal nerves. Through point 1, it is necessary to infiltrate anew under the aponeurosis of the external oblique a strip ending at two points situated, respectively, within and externally to the hernial ring; using approximately 20 mils of the weak solution. Through wheal No. 2, 10 mils of the solution are injected in a fan-shaped area to the line of the cord; the needle should strike the pubic bone. Through the same point, 10 mils are next injected in the inguinal canal itself along the cord. Finally, subcutaneous infiltration is conducted following the lozenge-shaped figure shown in the illustration, approximately 100 mils of the weak solution—½ per cent.—being used altogether (Figs. 140 and 141).

IRREDUCIBLE OR STRANGULATED INGUINAL HERNIA.

Four wheals are made as indicated in Fig. 142. Through wheal No. 1 one injects, as before, against the iliac bone, and continues toward wheals Nos. 2 and 3, injecting under the aponeurosis. Next, two deep injections are made through points 2 and 3. While the left hand pushes laterally inward and outward the hernia mass, the needle is inserted as far as the pubis, under the

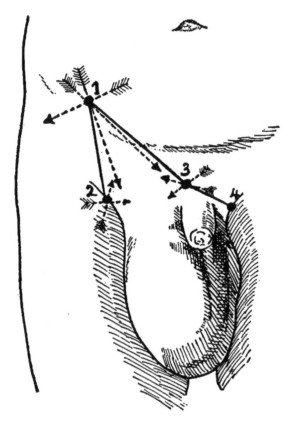

Fig. 142.—Lines of infiltration for inguinal hernia. (*Sourdat.*)
For irreducible or strangulated hernia.

hernia, and injection made deeply in the canal through points 2 and 3 along the neck of the sac. Finally, a subcutaneous injection between the points 1-2-3 and 2-3-4, is made. For a large hernia 150 mils of the weak solution may be used.

We prefer in such cases the paravertebral form of anesthesia, which deals with the nerves supplying the cord. The procedure just described, however, will likewise give satisfaction (Figs. 142 and 143).

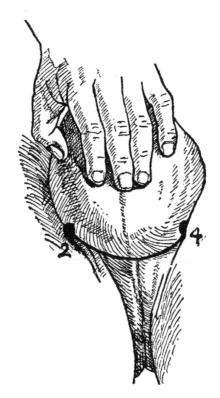

Fig. 143.—Anesthesia of the scrotum for irreducible hernia. (*Sourdat.*) Subcutaneous infiltration of the root of the scrotum through a crown of wheals.

FEMORAL HERNIA.

The nerve supply in femoral hernias is essentially that of the inguinal region. The anesthetic procedure, therefore, is almost the same:

Four dermal wheals are made. Point 1 occupies the same place as in inguinal hernia, viz., two finger-breadths within the anterior superior iliac spine. Points 2 and 3 are within and out-

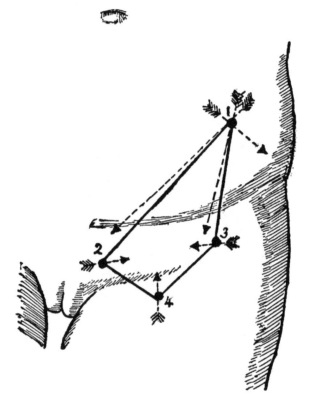

Fig. 144.—Reducible femoral hernia. The deep injections (arrows) and subcutaneous circuminfiltration are made through wheals 1, 2, 3, and 4.

side of the hernia, respectively, and at both ends of the intended femoral incision, parallel to the femoral arch. Point 4 is below the hernial mass.

One starts with the intramuscular injections at point 1. Through this one injects under the aponeurosis up to and outside of the neck. Then,

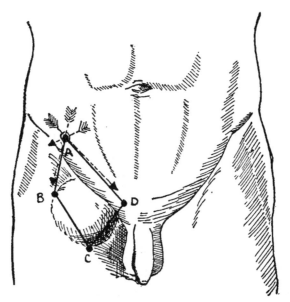

Fig. 145.—Irreducible femoral hernia. (*Pauchet.*) A fan-shaped intramuscular injection is made through point *A*. Infiltration of a subcutaneous band surrounding the hernial tumor and neck is conducted through points *A*, *B*, *C*, and *D*.

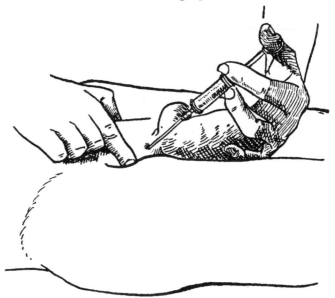

Fig. 146.—Anesthesia of the hernial sac and testicle by infiltration of the cord. Injection of the cord in the inguinal canal.

under the femoral arch through point 4, 10 mils of the solution are infiltrated around the neck, and very close to it.   Finally, subcutaneous infiltration is effected.   The femoral arch is anesthetized by this procedure.   If it be necessary to combine an inguinal incision with the high femoral incision, the anesthesia will be sufficient for the purpose. We have never been compelled to give ethyl chloride to the patient during the liberation of the intestine.   When, however, in a stout patient, we contemplated radical cure of a femoral hernia through the inguinal route, the patient complained somewhat while we were working deeply, showing that the anesthesia had been incorrectly instituted.

OPERATIONS UPON THE KIDNEY.

Nephrectomy is another operation for which regional anesthesia is indicated.   This method saves the renal tissue in the same way as it does the hepatic.   The anesthesia, moreover, is complete.   The lateral position of the subject can be maintained without the help of an assistant, the patient's voluntary aid being sufficient.   Decortication of the kidney and the ligation of the pedicle are painless.   We employ unilateral paravertebral injection of the six lower intercostal and of two lumbar nerves.   When once familiar with the technique, one no longer finds it necessary to have the patient inhale any additional anesthetic at the time of decortication of the kidney.

OPERATIONS UPON THE BILIARY PASSAGES.

It is advantageous to perform these without ether or chloroform, the harmful action of which upon the hepatic cells is well known. Our first operations under paravertebral anesthesia were done upon patients suffering from chronic jaundice,—of two months' standing in one instance (pancreatic tumor) and in another, six months (former lithiasis, with acute obstruction of the ductus choledochus). The post-operative course was devoid of complications, and the operations were absolutely painless, even in the second case, rendered difficult by multiple, long-standing adhesions. Since then all of our hepatic and biliary operations have been conducted under paravertebral anesthesia.

Right-sided paravertebral infiltration of the six lower intercostals and first two lumbar are required for the purpose. Here, as in the case of the kidney and other similar operations, one is struck by the *frequent diminution of post-operative pain* in the succeeding twenty-four hours. The method allows of the performance of cholecystectomy. Vertical or transverse incisions may be employed provided they do not cross the median line. The cushion placed under the chest may be a cause of suffering, which is obviated by a previous injection of morphine.

CHAPTER VI.

ANESTHESIA OF THE GENITO-URINARY ORGANS AND RECTUM.

THE pelvic organs and external genitalia are supplied by the internal pudic nerve, the small sciatic, and the sacral and coccygeal plexuses, which anastomose with branches from the pelvic sympathetic.

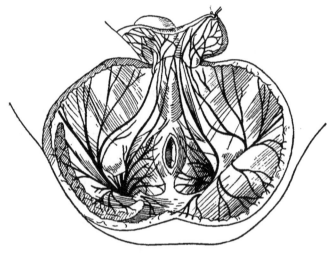

Fig. 147.—Nerve supply of the perineum in the male. (*Pauchet.*) Trunk of the internal pudic nerve and branches of the small sciatic.

The internal pudic nerve emerges from the pelvis through the great sciatic notch, winds around the external surface of the sciatic spine, traverses the ischio-rectal fossa, and gives filaments to the

(200)

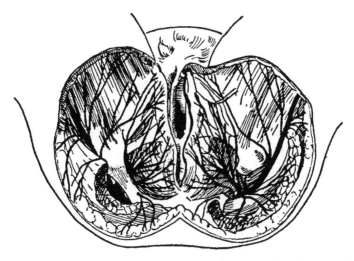

Fig. 148.—Nerve supply of the perineum in the female. (*Pauchet.*)   Internal pudic nerve and branches of the small sciatic.

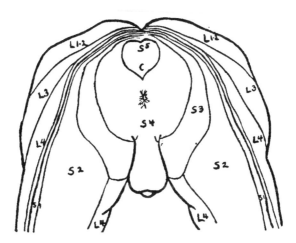

Fig. 149.—Sensory segments of the perineum corresponding to the last spinal pair. (*Pauchet.*)   The branches S indicate the sacral nerves, with the number of the foramen of emergence. The branches L are lumbar. The number is that of the corresponding segment. (See also Figs. 220 and 221.)

skin of the perineum, anus, posterior half of the
scrotum, penis, and vulva. The anterior half of
the scrotum and of the labia majora is supplied
by the genito-crural and the ilio-inguinal. The

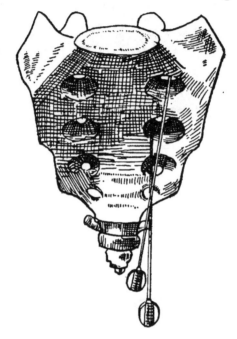

Fig. 150.—Pre-sacral anesthesia. (*Pauchet.*) To reach all
sacral foramina but the first, the needle is introduced between
the anus and coccyx and follows the anterior surface of the
sacrum to each foramen. To reach the first sacral foramen,
the needle is inserted at the same point but is pushed directly
through the tissues to reach the sacral brim When the bone
has been reached, the injection is made.

2d, 3d and 4th sacral pairs constitute the hypogastric plexus, and through it supply the bladder,
prostate, uterus, rectum, and pelvic peritoneum.

Regional anesthesia for the above operations is
simple and easy of application, and the various
regions involved and methods of treatment are

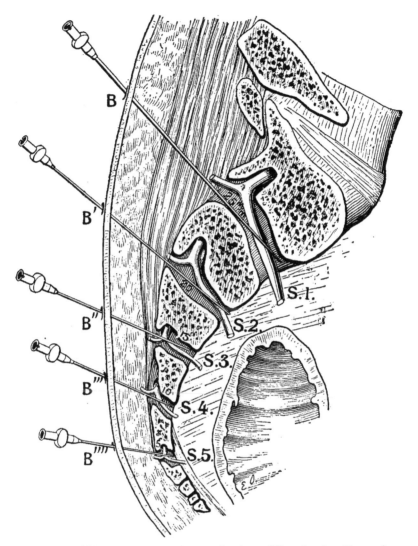

Fig. 151.—Trans-sacral anesthesia. (*Pauchet.*) Note the depth to which the needle *B* penetrates to reach the posterior foramen *S1*. On the contrary *B* finds the orifice *S5* immediately beneath the skin. The needle penetrates approximately 25 millimeters to reach the first sacral foramen, 20 for the second, 15 for the third, and 10 for the fourth, and should be driven about 1 centimeter into each canal in order to reach the anterior as well as the posterior division of the nerve. It is well to introduce the index finger into the rectum in order to be certain that the point of the needle is not penetrating the rectal wall.

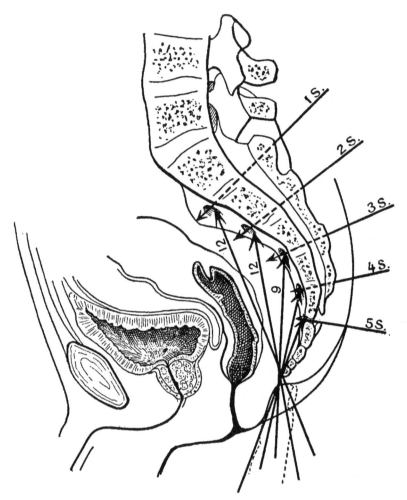

Fig. 152.—Pre-sacral and trans-sacral anesthesia. (*Pauchet.*)
The first of these procedures is indicated in the obese and the
second in thin subjects. In the latter the bony landmarks are
more easily found. Note the direction followed by the pre-
sacral needle for each foramen. The first four anterior arrows
reach the foramina 5, 4, 3, and 2. The needle point should be
kept in constant contact with the concavity of the sacrum, and
should always be parallel to the middle line of this bone. The
arrow destined for *S1* aims directly at the superior strait of
the pelvis. As soon as it comes in contact with this, the needle
is at the sacral foramen *S1*. If injury of the rectum is appre-
hended, a finger should be inserted in it during the introduction of the needle.

fully shown in Figs. 147 to 158. In Fig. 152 are shown the two methods of application. In thin subjects the injections are made through the five sacral foramina. In stout subjects it is often easier to reach the sacral nerves by introducing the needle at a point between the rectum and the tip of the coccyx, and infiltrating the concavity of the sacrum with a 1 per cent. solution of pro-caine-adrenin.

ANTERIOR SACRAL (PRE-SACRAL) ANESTHESIA.

The patient is placed in the dorsal position, with the thighs flexed upon the abdomen. After proper preparation of the skin with iodine and alcohol, an intra-dermal wheal is formed at a point midway between the anus and the tip of the coccyx, thus permitting the introduction of the successive needles without pain.

Through the wheal thus formed a needle 9 centimeters long is introduced and with its point the inferior and outer border of the sacrum about 2 centimeters from the median line is found. The needle is now pushed forward, with its point in constant contact with the anterior face of the sacrum, for about 1 centimeter, which should bring the point to a level with the fifth sacral foramen. Five mils of a 1 per cent. solution are thereupon injected.

One then continues upward, parallel and at about 2 centimeters from the median line, keeping the needle point constantly in contact with the surface of the bone, at a distance of about 1½ to 2 centimeters from the point already injected, when it should be at the level of the fourth sacral foramen. Here again 5 mils of 1 per cent. solution are injected. Then, with the needle in contact with the bone and always about 2 centimeters from the median line, one proceeds about 1½ to 2 centimeters higher up to the third foramen, where 5 mils should again be injected. In the same manner the needle is pushed upward a fourth time to the second foramen, where the same amount of solution is again injected. The needle is next drawn back to the starting point and the same manipulation repeated on the opposite side of the median line, thus bringing under control both sets of nerves.

The first needle is now replaced by one 12 centimeters long, the gloved finger placed in the rectum, and the needle introduced at the same point. Instead of following the surface of the bone, however, one next pierces directly upward to a depth of 9 to 10 centimeters, and with the finger in the rectum aiding as a guide, aims to strike the upper part of the sacrum as it tilts forward. At this depth, about 2½ centimeters from the median line and against the bone, the first sacral foramen is attained. Five mils of solution are injected and the procedure repeated on the opposite side. The last injection is an extra precaution. As a rule it is not needed, complete anesthesia of the parts being secured by injection of the other four pairs.

Anesthesia Through the Sacral Foramina— Trans-sacral Anesthesia.

The patient is placed in the extended posture and face down upon the table.   With the aid of

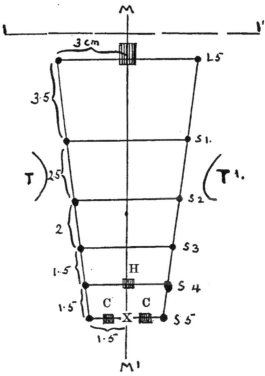

Fig. 153.—Location of the posterior sacral foramina. (*Pauchet.*) *MM'*, middle line of the body. *V*, spinous process of the 5th lumbar vertebra. *I-I'* lines joining the iliac crests. *TT'*, postero-inferior spines of the ilia. *H*, fourth sacral spinous process. *CC*, sacral cornua. *X*, sacral hiatus.

a dermographic pencil, a line is drawn from the crest of one ilium to that of the other (Fig. 156, CC).   The relationship of the posterior superior spines of the ilia is shown at *EE*.   The sacral cornua, *BB*, are now found and marked. From top to bottom a line is drawn directly over

the median line from D to A.   A point 4 centimeters on each side from the median line, on the
line CC, is marked.   This point is connected on

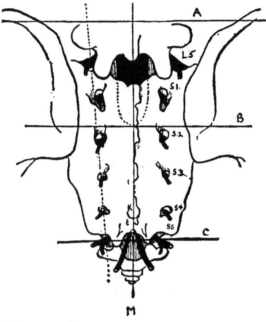

Fig. 154.—Posterior surface of the sacrum, showing the
posterior sacral foramina and sacral nerves. (*Pauchet.*) *A*,
the interiliac line. *B*, line joining the two postero-inferior
iliac spines. *M*, line joining the two middle spinous processes.
C, horizontal line passing through the two sacral cornua at
the level of the sacral foramen, *S5*. The oblique line corresponds to the situation of the sacral foramina; it is located
25 millimeters from the middle line at the level of the two sacral cornua. Note that the lumbo-sacral space, through which
spinal anesthesia may be induced (Le Filliâtre) is at the middle of the interval that separates *A* from *B*. *K*, point corresponding to the fourth sacral spinous process. *S4* is situated
1 centimeter outside of *K*.

each side by a line drawn downward to the
point B. ˙ The line passes directly over the five
sacral foramina.   Commencing at the top, the first
foramen is found on this line directly opposite the

tip of the spinous process of the fifth lumbar
vertebra (Fig. 153).

At a point 3½ centimeters below on the same
line will be found the second foramen. Two and
one-half. centimeters further down is the third; 2
centimeters down is the fourth, and 1½ below
this is the fifth. The first is about 35 mm. from
the median line; the second, 30; the third, 25; the
fourth, 20, and the fifth, 15 mm.

Technique of the Injections.—The spine is
painted with iodine, which is then removed with
alcohol. With a fine needle five dermal wheals
are injected on each side of the median line at
points overlying the sacral foramina. One com-
mences at the top with a needle 9 centimeters
long; if it does not at once enter the foramen the
operator will readily find the opening by feeling
about with the point of the needle. The latter
should penetrate to a depth of about 25 mm. for
the first foramen; 20 mm. for the second; 15 mm.
for the third; 10 for the fourth, and 5 for the
fifth. Five mils of a 1 per cent. solution are to
be injected at each opening.

In feeling about with the point of the needle,
seeking the opening, the operator will suddenly
sense the absence of resistance as the needle enters the foramen, and at the same moment the
patient is likely to complain of a disagreeable sensation in the abdomen or legs which is proof that
the nerve has been struck. After fifteen minutes
the operation can be begun. The anesthesia lasts
from one and one-half to two hours.

14

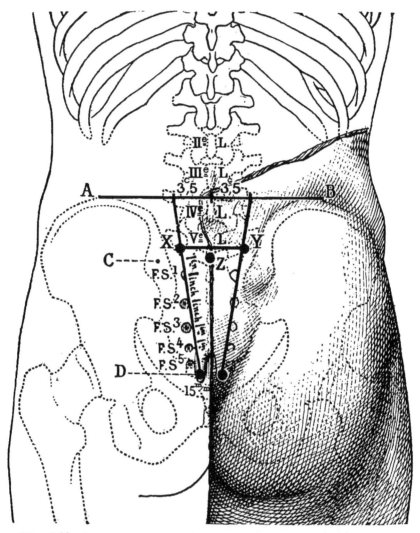

Fig. 155.—Trans-sacral anesthesia of the pelvic organs and pelvic peritoneum. The two iliac crests should be felt for and the line *AB* marked out. The prominent postero-inferior spine is at C, and the sacral cornu at *D* (sacro-coccygeal articulation). C is placed slightly too high in the sketch. The reader will notice at his right the prominent postero-inferior spine exactly outside of the sacral foramen, *S2*. *S5* is exactly outside of the sacral cornu. *S2* and *S1* are separated by the width of the thumb, as are also *S2* and *S3*. *S4* and *S5* are separated by the width of the little finger; the former corresponds to the summit of the sacral hiatus. The sacral foramina are situated on a line starting from the sacral cornu 15 millimeters from the median line and ending at the line *AB*, 35 millimeters from the median line. *Z*, the lumbosacral hiatus, is at the same distance from *S2* and from *AB*. *XY* corresponds to the 5th lumbar. These landmarks are utilized in posterior sacral anesthesia as well as in spinal anesthesia.

Sacral injections anesthetize the labia, prostate, bladder, rectum, anus, uterus, and skin of the posterior surface of the thigh. We use this method to do prostatectomies, extirpation of the

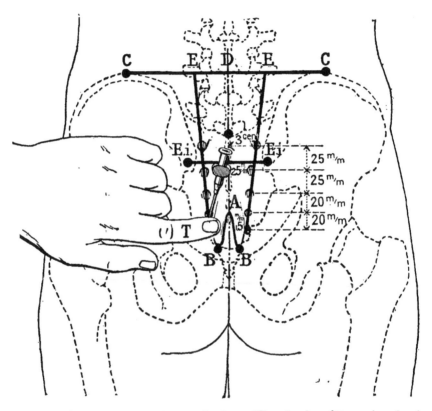

Fig. 156.—Trans-sacral anesthesia. (*Pauchet.*) (Posterior landmarks:· Fig. 155). *CC*, inter-iliac line. *EB, BE*, a trapezoid figure the base of which measures 8 centimeters and the summit, 3 centimeters. The points *BB* correspond to the sacrococcygeal articulation and the cornua of the sacrum; they are located 15 millimeters from the midline. The 5th sacral foramen is situated immediately outside of them. *Ei*, postero-inferior iliac spine (here shown a little high). The black dot between *D* and the line *Ei, Ei* should be at equal distance from *D* and *Ei, Ei, i.e.*, in the lumbo-sacral space or area of election for lumbar puncture. The distance separating each sacral foramen from the midline is also shown. The finger, *T*, shows that there is a finger-breadth of distance between the sacral foramina. The needle is entering foramen No. 4.

rectum, radical cure of prolapsus uteri, all vesical operations, curettage of the uterus, and catheterization of the ureters in man (for tuberculosis, cystitis, etc.), but the parietal peritoneum is not sufficiently anesthetized to permit of a hysterectomy. (See also Figs. 220 and 221, p. 282.)

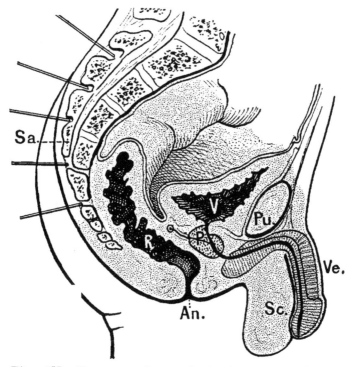

Fig. 157.—Trans-sacral anesthesia in man. (*Pauchet.*) This permits of operating upon a cancer of the rectum, hemorrhoids, prostatic adenoma, tumor of the bladder, amputation of the penis, etc.

OPERATIONS UPON THE BLADDER.
SUPRAPUBIC CYSTOSTOMY.

To perform a suprapubic cystostomy, the transsacral and hypogastric forms of anesthesia combined are necessary. For a cystostomy a lozenge is made the long axis of which corresponds to the lower half of the distance between the umbilicus and the pubis. The skin and muscles are infiltrated with the weak solution. The bladder is not anesthetized; but infiltration of the space of Retzius sufficiently diminishes its sensibility. One

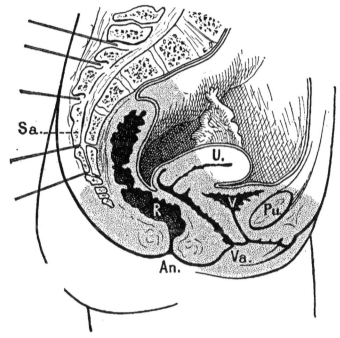

Fig. 158.—Trans-sacral anesthesia in woman. (*Pauchet.*) The gray area shows the region anesthetized by injection of the sacral nerves (pelvis and perineum). This enables the surgeon to operate upon cancer of the rectum, hemorrhoids, prolapsus uteri, or cystocele, and the obstetrician to use forceps without pain.

should add an intravesical injection of 50 mils of a ½ per cent. solution, allowed to remain during fifteen or twenty minutes for a simple section and vesical exploration. The bladder is rendered en-

tirely insensitive by the sacral injections, but the
abdominal wall must be infiltrated in addition before it is incised.

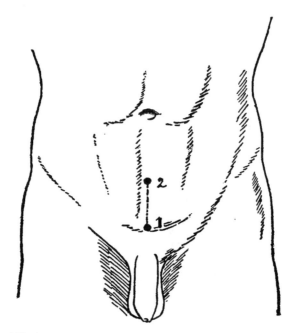

Fig. 159.—Suprapubic cystostomy. (*Pauchet.*) The operator makes two wheals, 1 and 2; then infiltrates the subcutaneous cellular tissues for a thumb's width to the right and left, ·
and the two recti abdominis. Through wheal 1, he injects the
space of Retzius in order to desensitize the bladder.

Operations upon the Testicles and Scrotum.

The operator should first anesthetize the cord,
then make a ring of anesthesia about the base of
the scrotum, on both sides. A wheal is made
over the external abdominal ring. With the left
hand, the cord is held firmly over the pubis, a
needle detached from the syringe inserted, the cord

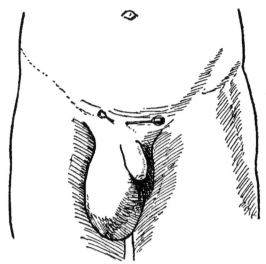

Fig. 160.—Anesthesia of the testicle. (*Pauchet.*) Infiltration of the cord by transfixion of it upon the pubis. In order not to miss the cord, the needle is pushed successively in two or three divergent directions.

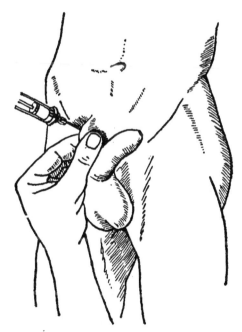

Fig. 161.—Anesthesia of the testicle. (*Pauchet.*) Infiltration of the cord. The latter is pinched between the fingers through the skin, raised between two fingers, and injected.

transfixed upon the pubis, then, after slight withdrawal of the needle, 5 mils of the weak solution injected; this infiltrates the cord. To make
certain, the maneuver is repeated and the cord
immobilized upon the pubis, transfixed, and infiltrated with 5 mils of the weak solution. Then,

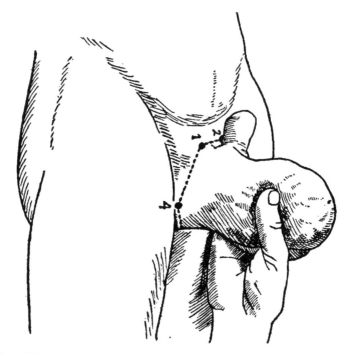

Fig. 162.—Operations upon the scrotum. (*Pauchet.*) A band
of subcutaneous infiltration circumscribes its base.

with the left index finger, the operator finds the external inguinal ring, introduces the needle from 6 to
9 centimeters into the inguinal canal, and injects
anew 10 mils of the weak solution.

To anesthetize the scrotum, the operator should
work all the way round its base, starting at the
lower surface of the penis, and, passing around,

infiltrate the subcutaneous tissue until he gets back to the starting point. He then passes in front of the perineum and in the genito-crural folds. The weak solution is sufficient; 50 mils, more or less, are required.

OPERATIONS UPON THE PENIS.

If it is desired to effect merely a dorsal incision of the prepuce, with simple section of the frenum,

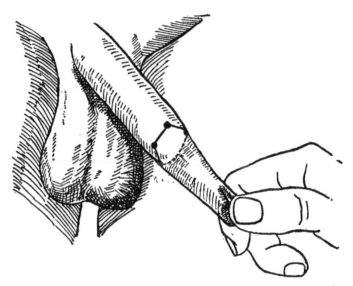

Fig. 163.—Anesthesia of the prepuce by a coronal injection. (*Pauchet.*)

the skin should be infiltrated in the median line by the "Reclus method" from the anterior aspect of the prepuce to the corona of the glans. One is thus enabled to slit the prepuce with scissors and suture the borders of the wound. A second injection being made at the level of the frenum, this may be split and one or two sutures taken

in it. We favor this simple operation, rather than
that of circumcision.

If the operator wishes to do an ordinary circumcision, amputate the penis, or operate upon a
hypospadias, it will be necessary for him to institute a total anesthesia of the penis in the following manner: A wheal is made at the right and
left of the root of the penis, where the cord

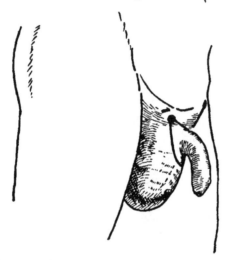

Fig. 164.—Anesthesia of the penis. (*Pauchet.*) Through
two wheals an injection is made at first deeply up to the roots
of the corpora cavernosa and the suspensory ligament, then
under the skin in circular fashion.

crosses over the horizontal ramus of the pubis.
Through this wheal the needle is introduced up to
the corpora cavernosa, under the suspensory ligament of the penis, and deeply around the penis.
Forty mils of a ½ per cent. solution of procaine-
adrenin are injected. This injection will anesthetize the urethra, corpora cavernosa, glans
penis, etc.

Operations upon the Posterior Urethra.

For suture of the urethra, urethrotomy, etc., a wheal is first made in front of the anus in the median line. Then, through this wheal, the vertical plane of tissue that separates the anus and rectum behind from the urethra, bulb, and prostate in front is infiltrated. The left index finger is placed in the rectum and with the right hand a 9-centimeter needle is taken and passed in in the median line, very high up between the prostate and rectum; the operator now injects while withdrawing it. He then begins anew, without wholly withdrawing the needle, and passes to the right and to the left, in order to infiltrate a space 9 centimeters high and 2 or 3 wide. This plane separates the rectum and anus behind from the prostate and urethra in front. All the subcutaneous cellular tissues and the muscles should be infiltrated.

Finally, it is necessary to infiltrate the plane of section corresponding to the incision in perineotomy for operations on the prostate. The operator may in this way go up as high as the neck of the bladder and the prostate with perfect anesthesia. Yet, anesthesia by the sacral foramina is in every way preferable.

Operations upon the Prostate.
PROSTATECTOMY.

A choice may be made from one of the four following methods of anesthesia:

1. Periprostatic infiltration through the bladder.

2. Periprostatic infiltration through the perineum.

3. Anterior sacral anesthesia.

4. Posterior trans-sacral anesthesia.

1. *Periprostatic Anesthesia Through the Bladder.*—(*a*) The operator begins by anesthetizing the abdominal wall, as for a cystotomy, then the space of Retzius. The simple infiltration of these tissues yields a satisfactory anesthesia. The injection must be carefully pushed into the entire thicknesses of the muscles, in order to be able to separate them without pain.

(*b*) For anesthesia of the prostate, the bladder having been opened, the operator takes a long curved needle (Legueu's) and passes through the mucosa of the bladder around the prostate, with the finger as guide. Approximately 150 mils of the weak solution of procaine-adrenin is used. Five or six minutes after this infiltration the operator may begin removing the prostate.

2. *Periprostatic Anesthesia Through the Perineum.*—The operator, after having infiltrated the abdominal wall as in the preceding method for a suprapubic section, must anesthetize the tissues between the two ischia, comprising the skin and soft parts situated between the urethra in front,

and the rectum and anus behind. This form of infiltration is useful for all operations upon the perineum (see Fig. 165).

To reach the prostate, the operator places his left index finger in the rectum in contact with the hypertrophied organ. With the right hand a 9-centimeter needle is introduced into the perineum and guided up toward the prostate by the aid of

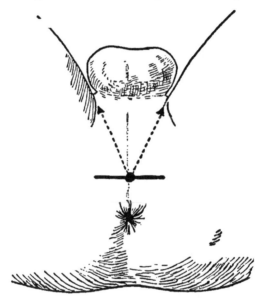

Fig. 165.—Anesthesia of the anterior portion of the perineum through a wheal in front of the anus. (*Pauchet.*)

a finger in the rectum. When the needle has attained the periprostatic region, 50, 60, or 80 mils of the weak solution of procaine-adrenin are injected.

3. *Anterior Sacral Method.*—This consists in infiltrating all of the concavity of the sacrum with a 1 per cent. solution. The needle should pass between the rectum in front and the sacrum be-

hind. The operator injects approximately 5 mils of procaine-adrenin opposite each one of the sacral foramina. It is unnecessary to inject the upper foramen (see Fig. 152 and detailed descriptions, including that of the trans-sacral method, at the beginning of this chapter).

4. *Trans-sacral Method.*—The operator must be experienced before such an anesthesia will prove perfectly satisfactory, but after some experience the *trans-sacral* method, which is *by long odds the best,* will be the one chosen.

With this procedure, very little of the anesthetic is required, and all that is needed in addition is the injection of the anterior abdominal wall.

OPERATIONS UPON THE VULVA AND VAGINA.

The posterior half of the vulva is supplied by the sacral nerves; the anterior half, by the ilio-inguinal and genito-crurals. If the operation indicated is one of minor importance, it is best to anesthetize the vulva directly. Three wheals are made, a middle one in front of the anus, and 2 lateral ones at the lower terminations of the labia majora. The soft tissues outside the labia majora are then infiltrated, thus completing the anesthesia (Fig. 166).

Where it is desired to anesthetize the vestibule of the vagina, the above method is not sufficient. One must infiltrate with the weak solution, following a frontal plane, in the manner already described for a perineotomy in the male. To infil-

trate the recto-vaginal septum, a finger should be
introduced in the vulva or rectum to guide the 9-
centimeter needle. One then infiltrates after Rec-
·lus's method, using 100 mils of the solution. After
this one may operate for a recto-vaginal fistula,
perform a perineorrhaphy, etc.

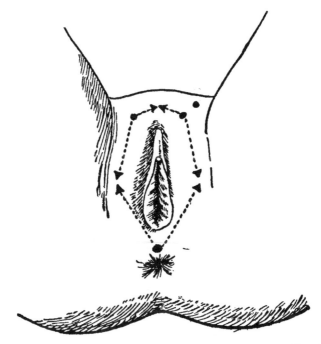

Fig. 166.—Anesthesia of the vulva and vestibule. (*Pauchet.*)

LIBERATION OF THE VAGINA AND OF THE UTERUS —PROLAPSE, COLPORRHAPHY, COLPOTOMY.

The preceding methods may be sufficient; this
simple infiltration, however, does not anesthetize
the pelvic floor. The vaginal vault should be infiltrated in addition. To do this, the cervix of the
uterus is brought down until it shows at the vulva;

a 9-centimeter needle is introduced into the anterior cul-de-sac, and 20 mils of solution injected between the bladder and the cervix (not under the mucous membrane). Another injection is now made under the urethral meatus, and this time right and left injections made on each side under the mucous membrane; 10 mils of solution are used. The cervix is pulled to the right and an injection made into the left lateral cul-de-sac, infiltrating the base of the broad ligament, using 15 mils. The operator begins anew on the right side, then introduces the 9-centimeter needle into the posterior cul-de-sac, between the vaginal mucous membrane and Douglas's cul-de-sac, injecting 20 mils. The uterus is now released and the perineum infiltrated as previously described. In all at least 200 mils are necessary.

A satisfactory anesthesia is obtained in a precise and simple way with the sacral method; but by this procedure no hemostasis is assured, while on the contrary, if infiltration is practised after Reclus's method, the operation is bloodless. In perineorrhaphy this is an advantage; from the anatomical point of view, however, the sacral method is more attractive, and we give it preference.

OPERATIONS UPON THE ANUS.

The trans-sacral procedure is very satisfactory in operations upon the anus. The perineal infiltration gives not only a good anesthesia, but also a perfect ischemia. All will agree that to extir-

pate hemorrhoids without the loss of a drop of
blood is ideal. For this reason, we give preference to the Whitehead operation, and infiltrate
at a distance around the anus and rectum when
the operation is practised, as upon a cadaver.

Four dermal wheals are made in a lozenge
form, one in front of the anus, two laterally, and

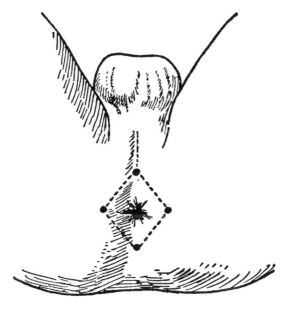

Fig. 167.—Anesthesia of the anal region through four
wheals circumscribing the anus and at some distance from it.
(*Pauchet.*)

the last behind, not too close, two finger-breadths
from the anal orifice (Fig. 167 and 169). Through
these four points all the injections, using ½ per
cent. solution, are made. Through the perineal
wheal, the needle is introduced, at first perpendicularly to the surface, and afterward in *a fan-
shaped* manner, right and left, each time 4 or 5

mils of the solution being injected deeply in the sphincter and under the skin. Through the lateral wheals fan-shaped injections are also made, parallel to the rectal walls, reaching the levator ani, and bathing the ischio-rectal fossæ, the sphincter, and the subcutaneous and submucous tissues (Fig.

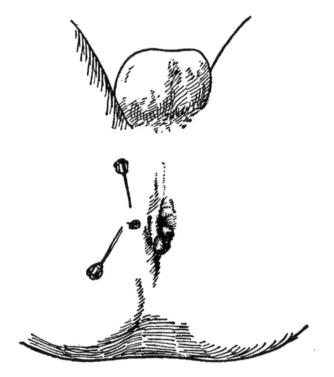

Fig. 168.—Radiating injections through the lateral wheal. (*Pauchet.*) The figure shows the three positions in which the needle should be placed in order to infiltrate the entire mass of tissue with quinine through a single wheal.

168). Finally, a mass of tissue is also infiltrated behind the anus and rectum, in fan-shaped fashion. The rectum is completely surrounded by the infiltration.

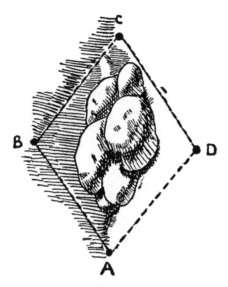

Fig. 169.—Radical cure of hemorrhoids by Whitehead's operation. (*Pauchet.*)   Through wheals *A, B,* C and *D,* a band
of tissue is infiltrated along the dotted lines.   Through the
same wheal deep radiating injections are then made in the
sphincter and adipose tissue of the ischio-rectal fossa, completely surrounding the ano-rectal cylinder.

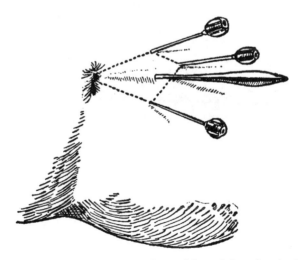

Fig. 170.—Peripheral infiltration with quinine for incision
of fistula *in ano.*   (*Pauchet.*)

At the close of the infiltration, when the latter
has been successful, *the sphincter is gaping.* In
a few minutes, dilatation, dissection and descent

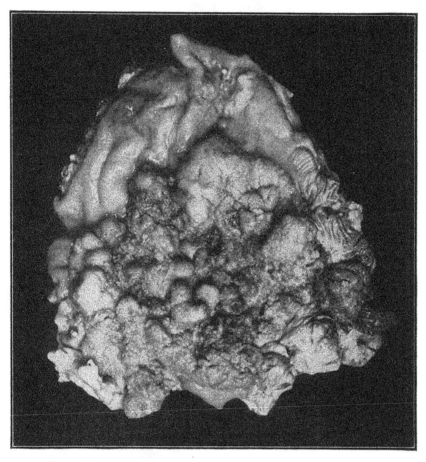

Fig. 171.—Anorectal segment laid open after extirpation.
(*Pauchet.*) Trans-sacral anesthesia is employed. The cancerous tumor forms a hollow cylinder.

of the mucosa, resection, and cauterization can be
effected without pain and without hemorrhage of
any account. According to the degree of stoutness of the patient, 50 or 100 mils of the solu-

tion are required.   Beginners should place a finger in the rectum to guide the needle.

Operations for fistula *in ano* may be done under the same method of infiltration.

We have often practised *total extirpation of the rectum,* with absolute anesthesia—always by the trans-sacral method.   Infiltration is not sufficient.   We practice the anterior or posterior method, according to the degree of stoutness of the patient.

CHAPTER VII.

ANESTHESIA OF THE EXTREMITIES.

REDUCTION OF FRACTURES OR DISLOCATIONS— QUÉNU'S METHOD.

IN 1907, Quénu recommended the use of local anesthesia for the reduction of fractures and dislocations.

The procedure consists in injecting in the vicinity of the fracture an anesthetic solution so that the bone ends are bathed with it, the seat of the fracture being thus rendered insensitive. The muscles simultaneously relax, and one may proceed without pain to dress the wound, examine the parts, reduce, practice radioscopy, etc. For dislocations, the injection is made into the synovial sac, then about the dislocated articulation and the insertion of the muscles surrounding it. The previously rigid limbs become supple and mobile, muscular contractions cease, and reduction becomes easy and painless. A 1 per cent. or ½ per cent procaine-adrenin solution is injected, according to the stoutness of the patient.

It will not be necessary to describe the procedure for every type of fracture or dislocation, the technique of the injection being practically the same in all. The procedure is easy and devoid of risk if a fine needle is used. A point at which the skin is not distended, contused, or trau-

(230)

matized in any way should be selected.   In juxta-
articular fractures,   the fracture   and   the   joint

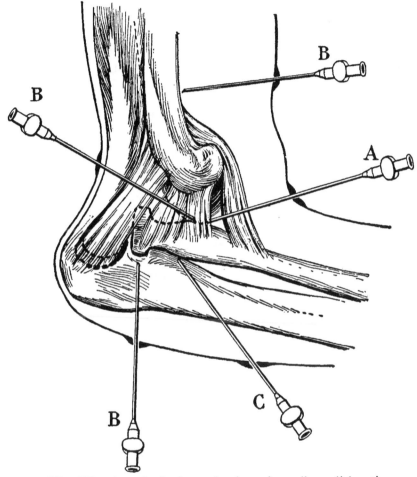

Fig. 172.—Anesthesia for reduction of an elbow dislocation.
(*Pauchet.*)   The quinine-urea solution is injected in the synovial sac of the articulation and infiltrates the insertions of the
muscles about the joint.

should be simultaneously injected.   In the lower
extremities this is the procedure of choice.   In the
upper, one may, with experience, instead, anesthetize the brachial plexus.

UPPER EXTREMITY.

The upper extremity as a whole, below the shoulder, receives its sensory supply from the brachial plexus, which becomes united beyond the scaleni into a single, comparatively narrow, cord. The upper intercostal nerves contribute in supply-

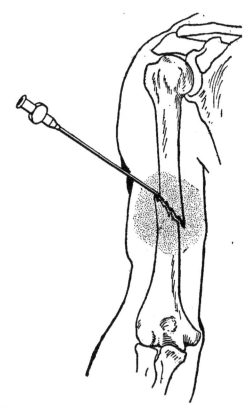

Fig. 173.—Anesthesia for fracture of the humerus. (*Pauchet.*) The needle is introduced at the site of fracture and quinine-urea solution injected throughout the region.

ing the axilla with sensation and also furnish a portion of the sensibility of the skin of the inner surface of the arm. The skin of the shoulder region is supplied by filaments from the supraclavicular branches of the cervical plexus.

ANESTHESIA OF THE BRACHIAL PLEXUS BY WAY OF THE AXILLA—HIRSCHEL.

The arm is extended in strong abduction (Fig. 174). With the left hand fixing the axillary artery, the needle is introduced high up as far as possible under the pectoralis major, following the longitudinal axis of the arm. The injection is begun during the introduction of the needle in order to push aside and avoid wounding the blood-

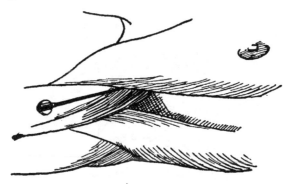

Fig. 174.—Infiltration of the brachial plexus by way of the axilla. (*Pauchet.*) Below the inferior border of the pectoralis major, with the arm abducted, the needle is introduced toward the nervous trunks, in a direction parallel with the axis of the arm.

vessels. With a few syringefuls of the solution, the median nerve is blocked above, and the ulnar further anteriorly. To reach the radial nerve, one must penetrate more deeply under the artery, almost to the height of the insertion of the pectoralis major. The artery is there surrounded with injections, and with proper caution injury to it or to the vein is avoided. Thirty or 40 mils of the 2 per cent. solution are used.

ANESTHESIA OF THE BRACHIAL PLEXUS BY THE SUPRACLAVICULAR ROUTE—KULENKAMPFF.

The location of the plexus is well shown, within by the subclavian artery, the pulsations of which can easily be felt; below, by the first rib, and in front, by the clavicle. Figure 175 shows the direction of the first rib, the supraclavicular region being seen in profile. It ascends behind

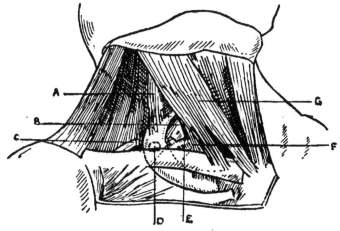

Fig. 175.—Blocking the nerve trunks of the upper extremity. (*Pauchet.*) *A*, scalenus posticus. *B,* apex of the pleura. C, omo-hyoid. *D*, point where the wheal should be made. *E*, subclavian artery. *F*, scalenus anticus. *G*, sterno-mastoid.

the clavicle and at a right angle, and is an important landmark, for it indicates the extreme point of penetration of the needle. The dermal wheal should be made at about the middle of the clavicle, where the first rib crosses it. The arch of the subclavian artery should be identified; it also crosses the clavicle at about its middle. Beyond lies the apex of the pleura, hidden by the plexus. Still further, at the external border of the sterno-cleido-mastoid, will be noticed the scalenus anticus, as well as the omo-hyoid, ascending obliquely from the first rib, and which has been divided, in order the better to show the course of the rib. Figure 176 shows the parts as they present themselves after removal of the skin and

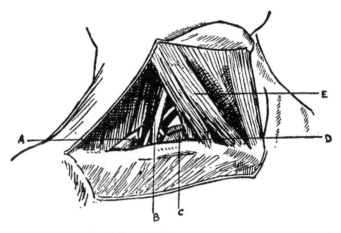

Fig. 176.—Anesthesia of the upper extremity. (*Pauchet.*)
A, omo-hyoid. *B*, brachial plexus. *C*, subclavian artery. *D*, scalenus anticus. *E*, sterno-cleido-mastoid.

the superficial and deep fascia. The transversalis artery of the neck is seen crossing the nerve trunks closely superimposed. Figure 177 and those following show the direction the needle should take. According to the more or less oblique direction of the first rib from the spine to the sternum, the needle, if prolonged, should reach the spinous process of the second or the third dorsal vertebra. On the other side are shown the plexus, the artery, the insertion of the scaleni, and finally, immediately below the clavicle, the crescent constituted by the nerves surrounding the artery. A needle introduced close to the artery and properly directed should pass through the middle of the nerve plexus. Almost always the pulsations of the artery will be transmitted to it. The narrowness of the interval between the scaleni is also apparent.

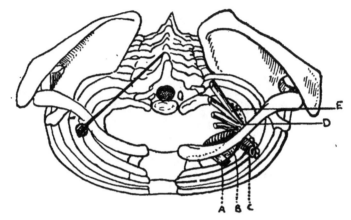

Fig. 177.—Anesthesia of the brachial plexus. (*Kulenkampff.*) Summit of the thorax. Direction of the needle to the left. To the right, relationship of the structures in the vicinity. *A*, subclavian vein. *B*, insertion of the scalenus antieus. *C*, subclavian artery. *D*, brachial plexus. *E*, insertion of the scalenus posticus.

TECHNIQUE OF THE INJECTION.

The patient should, if possible, be placed in the sitting posture (Fig. 178), and should be forewarned of the paresthesia radiating to the fingers that will occur when the needle touches the plexus, being requested to make known the moment when it appears. The subclavian artery is now slightly palpated with the finger. Its pulsations are often visible, especially on the right side. Just outside of the point where the artery descends behind the clavicle, with a fine needle, a wheal is made, which will correspond without exception to the middle of the clavicle.   The external jugular vein, often visible lower down, crosses the clavicle

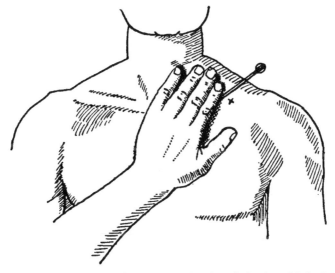

Fig. 178.—Supraclavicular anesthesia of the brachial plexus. (*Kulenkampff.*)   The left index finger locates and protects the subclavian artery.   Laterally to the artery and above the middle of the clavicle, (X), the needle is introduced in the direction of the spinous process of the third dorsal vertebra.

at the same point.   Through this wheal a fine needle 4 to 6 centimeters long is inserted and directed as if one desired to strike the spinous process of the second or third dorsal vertebra.   The plexus is superficially situated under the aponeurosis.   As soon as the needle strikes it, lancinating pains occur in the fingers supplied by the median, which is the most superficial, and the

radial, situated behind the median. If the first
rib is encountered at a depth of from 1 to 3
centimeters, the operator will· know that he has
missed and passed the plexus, as it is more superficially placed. If no paresthesia is produced, he

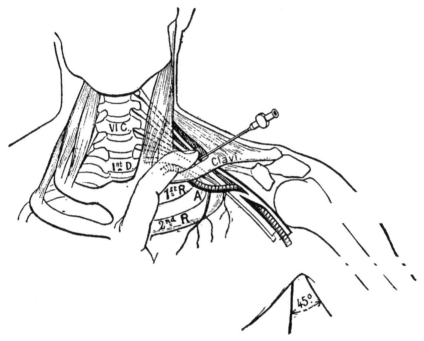

Fig. 179.—Blocking the brachial plexus. (*Pauchet.*) The
needle penetrates the skin above and close to the clavicle. It
traverses the plexus at the level of the clavicle and its point
touches the first rib. If the line of direction were prolonged it
would pass through the spinous process of the third dorsal
vertebra.

should try to provoke it by altering the position
of the needle. Very often, fear of wounding the
artery causes the operator to introduce the needle
too far out. If blood comes from the needle, it
is because a vein or artery has been pierced, and

its direction must be changed. The moment pares-thesia appears, the syringe is adapted to the needle and 10 mils of the 2 per cent. solution injected. If paresthesia is produced only in the

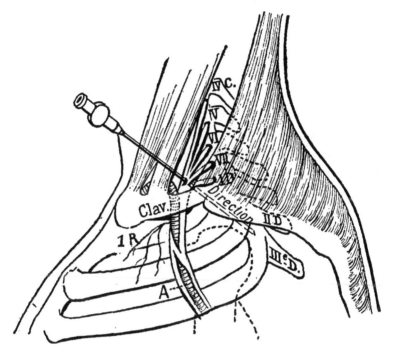

Fig. 180.—Blocking the brachial plexus. (*Pauchet.*) The needle is inserted just above the middle of the clavicle. The left index finger locates the pulsations of the artery and pushes it out of the way. Abduction of the arm to 45° (*Louis Bazy*) lifts away the artery and forms a curve with its concavity directed upward. The needle points toward the spinous process of the third dorsal vertebra. It passes through the plexus and strikes the first rib.

territory of the median, part of the solution should be injected some ·millimeters more deeply. The needle should be slightly displaced and 10 mils injected in the immediate vicinity. Under no circumstances should the injection be made before production of the paresthesia.

If unquestionable paresthesia has been obtained both in the territory of the median and that of the radial in from one to three minutes a complete motor and sensory paralysis will be established in the arm. ·Often one must wait from ten to fifteen minutes. If, at the end of this time, paralysis is not complete, 5 to 10 mils of the 4 per cent. solution may be injected. Success will then, however, be uncertain. After the injection, the tourniquet may be applied without pain. It is often useful, for after blocking of the brachial plexus the arm is habitually hyperemic, the vasomotors being paralyzed as after section of the nerves. The motor paralysis always reaches the circumflex nerve; but its territory is only hypoesthetized or uninfluenced. Other nerves, probably filaments from the supraclavicular, take part in the innervation of this region. ·The anesthesia lasts from one hour and a half to three hours.

ANESTHESIA OF THE BRACHIAL PLEXUS BY THE INFRACLAVICULAR ROUTE—LOUIS BAZY.

The brachial plexus assumes the shape of a fan, the axis of which is constituted by the seventh cervical nerve. The origin of this root is immediately below the anterior tubercle of the transverse process of the sixth· cervical vertebra (tubercle of Chassaignac). It is found on a level with the inferior border of the cricoid cartilage.

The tubercle of Chassaignac is, then, the first landmark.

After grouping themselves around the seventh cervical, the other branches of the cervical plexus

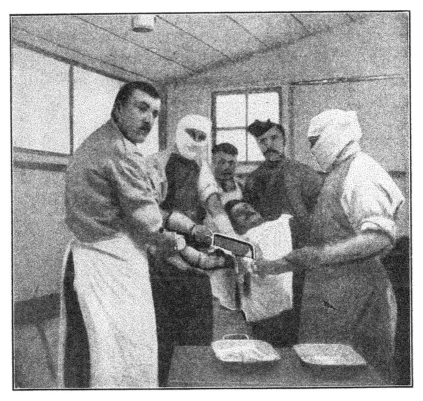

Fig. 181.—Infraclavicular anesthesia of the brachial plexus. (*Pauchet.*) Amputation of the arm performed on the Meuse at a spot 6 kilometers from the firing line. The operating room had been set up by the ambulance orderlies. Surgeon: Sourdat. Assistant: Louet, auxiliary physician. The patient is looking toward the camera.

become engaged in the space between the clavicle and the first rib, and afterward pass perpendicularly to the coracoid process. When the arm is abducted in such a way that the tangent passing

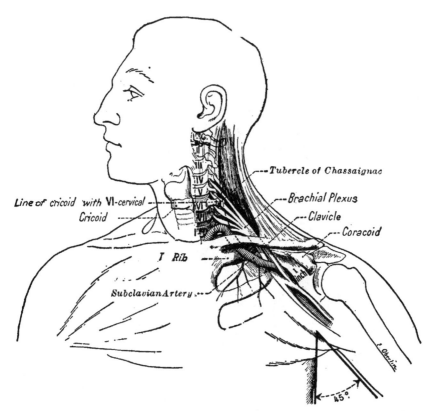

Line of cricoid with VI-cervical
Cricoid
I Rib
Subclavian Artery

Tubercle of Chassaignac
Brachial Plexus
Clavicle
Coracoid

45°

. Fig. 182.—Anesthesia of the brachial plexus by the infraclavicular route. (*Pauchet.*) Observe that the cricoid cartilage corresponds to the transverse process of the sixth cervical (tubercle of Chassaignac). This tubercle may be found by palpation, and the assistant should place his index finger there at the time of the injection. To the right, the coracoid process, and one fingerbreadth within it, the plexus. The operator introduces the needle here immediately below the clavicle and directs it toward the tubercle of Chassaignac. The arm having been abducted to 45°, the axillary artery is separated from the brachial plexus, drawn away by the two thoracic branches given off from its lower aspect. The artery rests on the first rib.

through the apex of the coracoid process strikes
the tubercle of Chassaignac, this line indicates exactly the direction of the brachial plexus, which
is situated one finger-breadth below it. This line
may be considered as the "line of anesthesia,"
and the coracoid process constitutes the second
landmark. In this position the arm forms with
the trunk an angle of 45° (Fig. 184). The axillary artery, held against the arm by its acromio-
thoracic branch, deviates from the brachial plexus,
describing a curve with its concavity upward. As
a result of this, the risk of wounding it is slight.

TECHNIQUE OF THE INJECTION.

The patient is placed upon the table, with his
spinal column resting upon a cushion in such a way
that his shoulders are arched, as though for ligation of the subclavian or axillary under the clavicle. The arm, hanging and abducted to 45°, renders the prominence of the coracoid more apparent, and the plexus more superficial.

The operator places himself on the side to be
operated upon, between the arm and the trunk.
He locates the apex of the coracoid and immediately within it, with the left index finger,
he depresses the soft tissues, as though wish-
ing to make more apparent the prominence of the
coracoid.

Meanwhile the assistant identifies the tubercle
of Chassaignac, over which he places his index
finger. The arm being abducted to 45°, the in-

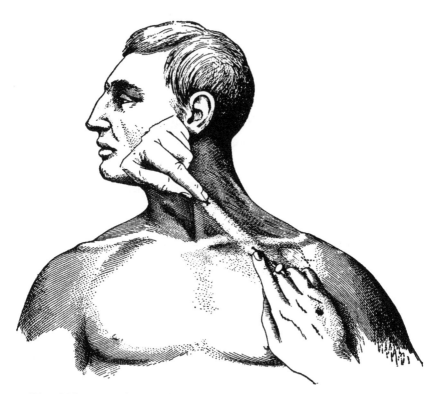

Fig. 183.—Anesthesia of the brachial plexus by the infraclavicular
route. (*Louis Bazy.*) The two hands show the "line of anesthesia."
The finger of an assistant is placed on the tubercle of Chassaignac;
the surgeon's finger, inside of the coracoid process, which is shown by
dotted lines. Here, within the finger tip, the needle enters immediately
below the clavicle and is directed toward the brachial plexus. It is
well to inject both upward, to the right, to the left, and deeply downward to be sure of reaching all the branches of the plexus.

dex finger of the operator and that of his assistant face each other, and the interval separating them marks the course of the plexus (Fig. 183). The line of anesthesia is now traced upon the skin with ½ per cent. procaine-adrenin solution.

A needle 9 centimeters long is introduced in the zone of infiltration, almost immediately below the clavicle. The needle is pointed in such a way that it grazes the posterior border of the bone. When the needle has passed slightly beyond the upper surface of the clavicle, 10 mils of 2.5 per cent. procaine-adrenin solution are injected. The arm is flexed as if one wanted to place it upon the chest. As a result of this maneuver the brachial plexus is relaxed and comes in front of the needle, when it can be directly penetrated and anesthetized.

OPERATIONS UPON THE HAND.

The technique of anesthetizing a finger by means of injections all round it under the skin of the first phalanx has been well described by Reclus and is too well known to require description anew. The adjacent parts of the metacarpus may, however, be anesthetized consentaneously with the finger.

ANESTHESIA OF A FINGER WITH THE ADJACENT PORTION OF THE METACARPAL.

Two wheals are made upon the dorsal surface of the interdigital space, corresponding to its in-

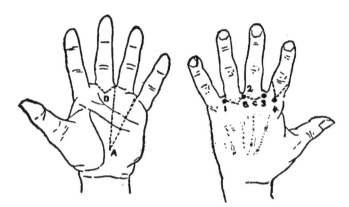

Fig. 184.—Landmarks for injection of the fingers. (*Pau-chet.*) The pyramid *A* shows the depth to which the needle is introduced, as illustrated in Fig. 187.

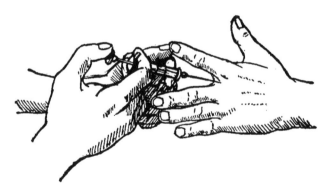

Fig. 185.—Manner of holding the syringe in infiltrating the palm by injection into the interdigital spaces.

ternal and external borders (Fig. 184). A ½ or
1 per cent. solution is freely injected under the
skin in the direction of points *A* or *D* in the
palm, and *B* or *C* in the back of the hand. Fig.
185 shows the course of the needle in an injection
in the palm through the interdigital space. The
operation should not be started until the anesthesia has reached the tip of the finger.

DISARTICULATION OF THE MIDDLE FINGER—OPERA-
TION UPON THE THIRD METACARPAL BONE.

Four wheals are made (Fig. 186), two in the
interdigital spaces, and two metacarpal, over the

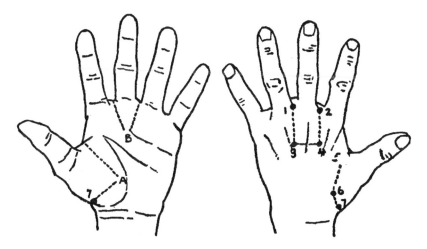

Fig. 186.—Anesthesia of the medius with the head of its
metacarpal; also anesthesia of the thumb with its metacarpal.
(*Pauchet.*)

interosseous spaces. The start is made at points
3 and 4. Fig. 189 shows a section of the metacarpus and the course followed by the needle.

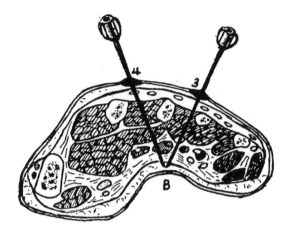

Fig. 187.—Infiltration of the palm of the hand through two injections from the dorsal aspect. (*Pauchet.*)

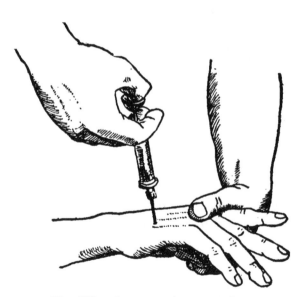

Fig. 188.—Same as the preceding.

The tip of the left index finger being placed in the patient's palm, the needle is introduced at 3 and 4, ·and the injection made perpendicularly through the interosseous space until the tip of the needle shows under the skin of the palm at *B* (Figs. 187 and 188). At each one of the two

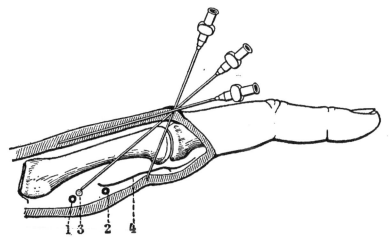

Fig. 189.—Anesthesia of a finger and its metacarpal bone. (*Pauchet.*)   Longitudinal section of an interosseous space showing the different directions that the needle should take. 1, deep palmar arch; 2, superficial palmar arch; 3, ulnar nerve; 4, palmar aponeurosis.

injections 5 mils of the ½ per cent. solution are used.   Next one infiltrates subcutaneously from points 1 and 2, in the palm toward point *B,* and upon the dorsum toward· 3 and 4.   Finally points 3 and 4 are united by a subcutaneous injection. In all, from 30 to 40 mils of the ½ per cent. solution are required.

DISARTICULATION OF THE THUMB WITH ITS METACARPAL.

The interosseous space is first injected, start-. ing from point 6 and introducing the needle to point *A* under the skin of the palm (Fig. 186). Owing to the thickness of the soft parts, 10 mils of the ½ per cent. solution are required. The next injection is made subcutaneously from points 5 and 7 toward the palm in *A,* upon the back of the hand from 6. About 50 mils of the ½ per cent. solution are used. The thenar eminence may thus be anesthetized without piercing the skin of the palm, which is very sensitive. The same procedure may be followed for the fifth metacarpal and finger.

ANESTHESIA OF SEVERAL FINGERS WITH THEIR METACARPALS.

Injections made at points 1, 2, and 3 (Fig. 190) anesthetize the second and third fingers. From point 2 the injection is pushed in the interosseous space against point *A,* and from points 1 and 3 in the palm toward point *A.* On the back of the hand one infiltrates under the skin toward point 2. Injections made at 4, 5, and 6 anesthetize the third and fourth fingers. Portions of the metacarpus may be, as desired, circumscribed in the anesthetized territory, according as the points of entry 2 or 6 are placed nearer the fingers or the. wrist. About 50 mils of ½ per cent. solution are required.

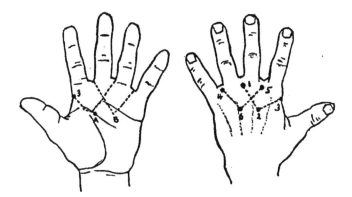

Fig. 190.—Anesthesia of two fingers with the heads of the metacarpal bones. (*Pauchet.*)

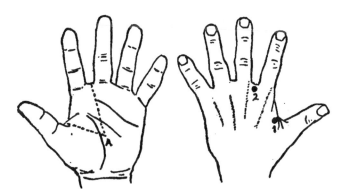

Fig. 191.—Anesthesia of one finger with the head of its metacarpal. (*Pauchet.*) Injections are made along the dotted lines through wheals at 1 and 2, circumscribing the region to be operated upon.

ANESTHESIA OF THE SOFT PARTS OF THE PALM.

Any portion of the palm may be anesthetized by employing the same technique as already des-

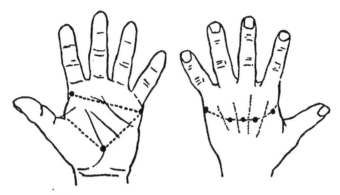

Fig. 192.—Anesthesia of a portion of the palm of the hand. (*Pauchet.*)

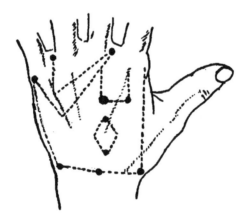

Fig. 193.—Lines of infiltration for minor operations upon the dorsal aspect of the hand. (*Pauchet.*)

cribed for anesthesia of the thenar and hypothenar eminences, *e.g.,* in disarticulation of the thumb. The needle should, however, always be entered upon the borders of the hand and upon the dorsal aspect of the interosseous spaces (Fig. 192). If it is desired to anesthetize the palm above the index finger (Figs. 191, 193), the wheals should be made at points 1 and 2. Through these two points, free injections are made toward point A in the palm, using 30 to 40 mils of the ½ per cent. solution. In the case of phlegmons of the hand, one should not inject in the vicinity of the affected parts, but resort instead to anesthesia of the brachial plexus.

ANESTHESIA OF THE SOFT PARTS OF THE BACK OF THE HAND.

In anesthesia instituted for the treatment of wounds or for the extirpation of ganglions, cysts, and other tumors, the field of operation is surrounded with a ½ per cent. solution. Fig. 193 shows the manner in which the infiltration should be conducted in different cases. All that is necessary is to surround three sides of the field in the form of a U, since the nerves descend from the forearm exclusively. The anesthesia reaches the periphery by reason of the injection of three sides and in some cases extends beyond it below the field of operation. If the injections be made first under the tendons, and then under the skin, the anesthesia will include tissues beneath the fascia.

ANESTHESIA OF THE ULNAR NERVE
AT THE ELBOW.

The ulnar nerve is ordinarily palpable above the epitrochlea, where it can be made to roll under the finger. In anesthesia it is fixed with the thumb and index finger of the left hand and the needle is pushed up to it through the subcutaneous tissues and fascia. The moment the nerve is touched, the patients will feel and complain of

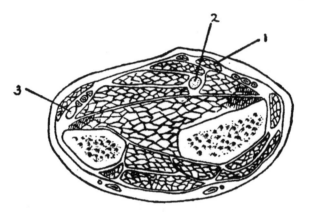

Fig. 194.—Section of the forearm above the wrist. (*Pauchet.*)
1, Palmaris longus. 2, Median nerve. 3, Ulnar nerve.

the same tingling as is experienced when the nerve is compressed. The solution is then injected. It should be noted that in many patients the ulnar nerve, when the arm is flexed, is situated not behind but in front of the epitrochlea, and passes behind only when the forearm is in extension. Anesthesia follows very quickly after the injection and involves the little finger, the hypothenar eminence, the ulnar border of the hand, and the fifth metacarpal. For disarticulation of the little finger and other operations in this region, there is no simpler procedure (Figs. 195 and 196).

ANESTHESIA OF THE ENTIRE HAND.

The hand receives from the forearm the ulnar, median and interosseous nerves, which are all

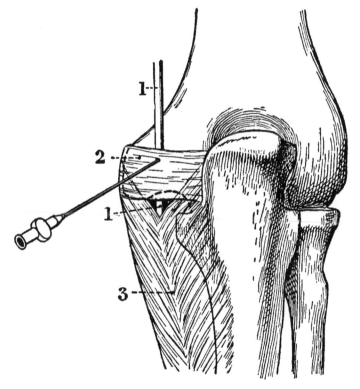

Fig. 195.—Anesthesia of the ulnar nerve. (*Pauchet.*) The nerve trunk is infiltrated in the depression between the epitrochlea and the olecranon process. 1. Ulnar nerve. 2. Fibrous arch. 3. Flexor carpi ulnaris.

three subfascial, together with the endings of the radial, which are subcutaneous. Fig. 198 presents a perpendicular section of the forearm above the

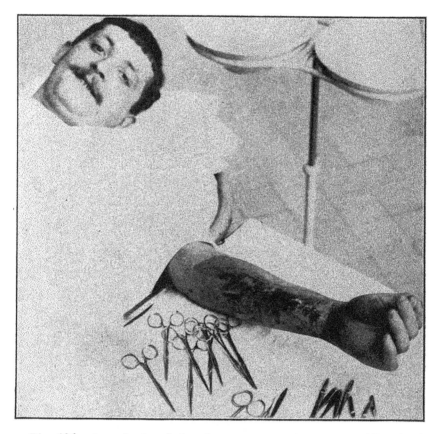

Fig. 196.—Anesthesia of the ulnar nerve at the elbow. (*Pauchet.*)
Anesthesia has been induced by means of an injection of strong procaine-adrenin solution in the depression between the epitrochlea and
the olecranon, as well as by a bracelet of subcutaneous infiltration at
the bend of the elbow. Suture of the ulnar nerve has been completed. The dissection of the nerve has been effected without any pain.
The wound is sutured with silkworm gut.

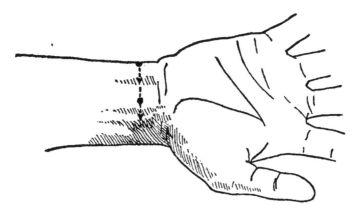

Fig. 197.—Points of introduction of the needle to reach the median and ulnar nerves above the wrist. The needle is pointed and the injections made in the direction of the arrows.

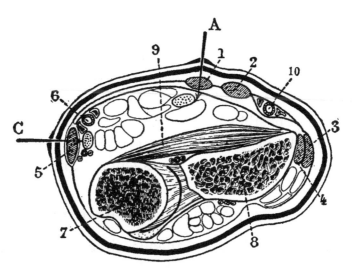

Fig. 198.—Anesthesia of the hand. (*Pauchet.*) Transverse section of the wrist at the level of the inferior radiocarpal articulation. Note the bracelet-like black line of subcutaneous infiltration. The arrows represent the deep injections intended for *A*, the median nerve, and C, the ulnar nerve. 1. Tendon of the palmaris brevis. 2. Tendon of the palmaris longus. 3. Tendon of the abductor longus pollicis. 4. Supinator longus. 5. Flexor carpi ulnaris. 6. Ulnar artery. 7. Ulna. 8. Radius. 9. Pronator quadratus. 10. Radial artery.

wrist, showing the direction in which the needle
should be pushed toward the median and ulnar
nerves.   To reach the median at this level, a
wheal is made on the ulnar side of the tendon
of the palmaris longus, and the needle pushed
through the fascia under this tendon.   The operator attempts to touch the nerve with the needle
point.   When the patient complains of shooting
pains, 5 mils of a 2 per cent. solution are injected.   Next, 5 mils of the same solution are
injected on the ulnar side of the forearm, above
the pisiform and beneath the tendon of the flexor
carpi ulnaris (Fig. 198).   Finally, one infiltrates
through two or three other points in ring fashion
around the forearm—under the skin, then upon
the dorsal surface under the fascia between the
tendons, and up to the interosseous ligament,
using 50 to 60 mils of a ½ per cent. solution.
Complete anesthesia of the whole hand is obtained in from ten to fifteen minutes.   This procedure is simpler than intravenous anesthesia.

OPERATIONS UPON THE FOREARM.

The skin and subcutaneous tissues of the forearm down to its lower third are exclusively supplied by long subcutaneous nerves that emerge
from under the fascia above the elbow.   Infiltration of a transverse band of subcutaneous tissue
on the forearm produces, therefore, an anesthesia
that becomes more or less extensive below the
level of injection, and when a circle of subcuta-

neous tissue above or below the elbow is infiltrated, the anesthesia extends on all aspects to the
lower third of the forearm.

For operations upon the skin of the upper two-
thirds of the forearm, the field of operation should
be surrounded by injections disposed in the shape

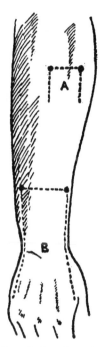

Fig. 199.—Anesthesia of the dorsal surface of the forearm and hand.   (*Pauchet.*)

of a U with its concavity directed downward,
using the ½ per cent. solution (Fig. 199). The
unilateral nerve supply of this region renders the
muscular injection unnecessary if the operation is
unilateral.

In the lower third the injection should also be
subfascial on account of the nerves that emerge

from within the forearm. Extensive areas upon
the lower third of the dorsal aspect of the forearm may be anesthetized as follows: Two injections are made upon the borders of the forearm, indicated by the bony ridge of the radius and
ulna (Fig. 199, *B*). With a long needle the soft
parts of the dorsal surface are infiltrated, beginning with the muscles, then the subcutaneous tissues transversally, with 40 or 50 mils of a ½
per cent. solution. From these two points the
subcutaneous infiltration descends to the wrist and,
if necessary, to the fingers. This procedure is
useful for the treatment of severe wounds of
the soft parts, the extirpation of tumors or cysts,
tuberculosis of the tendon sheaths, etc.

The procedure adapted for the lower half of
the anterior surface of the forearm differs slightly
by reason of the median and ulnar nerves. Two
injections are made upon the sides of the forearm,
and these are joined by infiltrating transversally
close to the bone and the interosseous ligament
at the start, and then in the subcutaneous tissue.
It is useless to try to infiltrate the muscles sep-
arately; this is almost impossible in any case, and
the median and ulnar are not blocked. If the
operative field is in the ulnar distribution, it is
best to inject this nerve at the elbow. If it is in
that of the median, then this nerve should be
anesthetized at the upper extremity of the incision.
Those well trained in anesthesia of the brachial
plexus will give this procedure the preference—
especially in phlegmons, operations on the bone,

amputations and interventions upon the upper half of the forearm, and in fact, in all operations of importance below the shoulder.

OPERATIONS UPON THE ELBOW.

A subcutaneous U-shaped infiltration with concavity downward, using 40 mils of a ½ per cent. solution, upon the dorsal surface of the elbow, and instituted through two wheals (Fig. 200), will permit of extirpation of the olecranon bursa. To suture a fractured olecranon, two additional injections are necessary, 3 and 4. One begins by injecting 20 mils of the ½ per cent. solution into

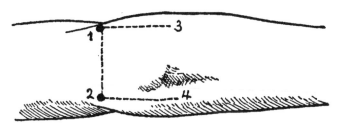

Fig. 200.—Anesthesia of the elbow region. (*Pauchet.*)

the articulation, below the external and internal condyles. Ten mils are injected under the tendon of the triceps in the muscles covering the olecranon, first inside and then outside, and finally the U-shaped subcutaneous injection is made. For an aseptic arthrotomy—as for the removal of foreign bodies—20 mils of the ½ per cent. solution are injected in the joint and the capsule and subcutaneous tissue infiltrated along the line of incision. To perform a resection or disarticulation, blocking of the plexus is necessary.

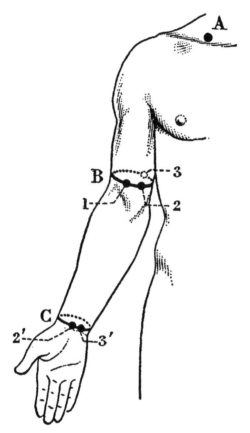

Fig. 201.—Anesthesia of the upper extremity. (*Pauchet.*)
A, Blocking of the brachial plexus, producing anesthesia of
the entire upper limb. *B*, Anesthesia of the forearm and hand.
C, Anesthesia of the hand only. The points 1, 2, 3, 2′ and 3′
are the wheals through which the subcutaneous bracelet of infiltration is made. The needle employed to infiltrate deeply the
nerve trunks is also introduced through them. 1, Anterior
branch of the radial nerve. 2 and 2′, Median nerve. 3 and
3′, Ulnar nerve.

Operations upon the Arm.

Local injections are here suitable only for superficial operations. A simple subcutaneous injection is insufficient by reason of the irregular and multiple branching of the nerves. A pyram-

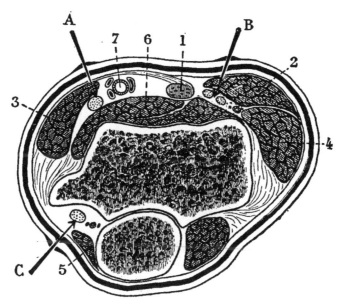

Fig. 202.—Anesthesia of the forearm and hand. (*Pauchet.*) Transverse section at the elbow. Note the bracelet of subcutaneous infiltration marked by a heavy black line. *A,* Deep injection to the median nerve. *B,* Deep injection to the radial. C, Deep injection to the ulnar. 1, Tendon of the biceps. 2, Supinator longus. 3, Pronator radii teres. 4, Extensor carpi radialis longus. 5, Flexor carpi ulnaris. 6, Brachialis anticus. 7, Brachial artery.

idal injection of the operative field is always required. To anesthetize the skin of the entire surface of the arm, as for Thiersch skin grafting, one infiltrates superficially all the subcutaneous tissue with a ½ per cent. solution, as for the thigh.

For extensive operations on the bones, amputations, etc., the plexus is injected above the clavicle (Fig. 181).

OPERATIONS UPON THE SHOULDER.

Large lipomas of the shoulder are easily removed after multiple infiltrations have been made

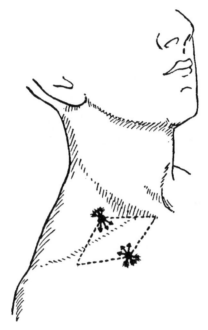

Fig. 203.—Suture of a fracture of the clavicle. (*Pauchet.*)
Through two injections the clavicle is surrounded, to any extent necessary, with the anesthetic solution.

all around them. The base of the tumor is
reached with long needles, and the injections are
connected with one another by bands of subcutaneous infiltration. A ½ per cent. solution is
used, and as much as 200 to 250 mils may be
injected.

Operations on the shoulder are performed after anesthesia of the plexus. For shoulder disarticulation, the plexus has first to be infiltrated, and then the subcutaneous tissues at the root of the shoulder up to the acromion and through the axilla. The ½ per cent. solution is used.

LOWER EXTREMITY.

It is difficult to anesthetize the lower extremity by local injections, as it receives its nerve supply from many different trunks. On the other hand, spinal anesthesia is very serviceable, and only a small amount of procaine-adrenin solution, 4 or 5 centigrams, need be used. The injection is made directly into the spinal canal of the lumbar region. In a large number of cases regional anesthesia is absolutely indicated, and succeeds admirably. Thus, all operations on the foot—reseetion, amputation, tenotomy, suture of the patella, operations for varicose veins, or on the inguinal lymphatics, etc.,—may be performed with complete anesthesia by the regional method. We give preference, however, to lumbar spinal anesthesia for all major operations, such as resection of the knee, resection of the hip, and amputation of the thigh. We probably practice three regional anesthesias to every spinal.

The *external cutaneous nerve* emerges from under the inguinal ligament immediately within the anterior superior iliac spine; it descends in an outward direction under the fascia lata; perforates the fascia, and supplies the skin. It can be reached two finger-breadths within and below the anterior superior spine (Figs. 204 and 205).

The technique is as follows: A dermal wheal

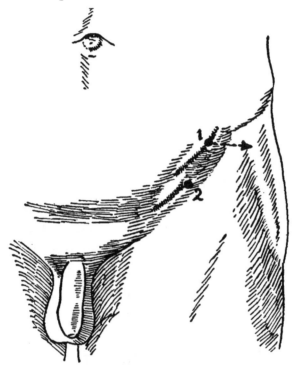

Fig. 204.—Injection of the external cutaneous nerve (1) and of the anterior crural nerve (2). (*Pauchet*.) 1, Point where the needle should be introduced to reach the external cutaneous; the injection is made in the direction of the arrow, beneath the fascia and skin. 2, Point of entrance of the needle, perpendicularly to the surface, to reach the anterior crural nerve.

is made and the subcutaneous connective tissue so injected as to make a transverse band 5 or 6 centimeters wide, parallel to Poupart's ligament. Five mils of the strong solution are then injected under the fascia, in the same direction as the sub-cutaneous infiltration. The middle of the infiltrated area should be situated two finger-breadths within and below the anterior superior spine.

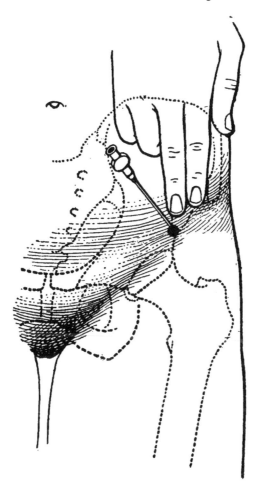

Fig. 205.—Anesthesia of the external cutaneous ·nerve. (*Pauchet.*) This nerve is reached at a· point two finger-breadths within and below the anterior superior spine of the ilium.

The *anterior crural nerve* is situated imme-diately outside of the femoral artery and is cov-·ered by a fibrous band (ilio-pectineus). With the left hand the operator locates the pulsations of the femoral artery and pushes the latter inward. The needle is then introduced immediately outside the artery, just below Poupart's ligament. Where it comes in contact with a solid band of fascia, the latter is pierced and 5 mils of the strong

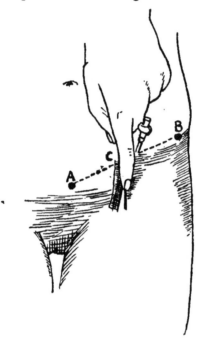

Fig. 206.—Anesthesia of the anterior crural nerve. (*Pauchet.*) *A*, Spine of the pubis. *B*, Anterior superior iliac spine. *C*, Point half way between the two. The femoral artery is located with the finger. The needle is inserted one finger-breadth outside of it to reach the anterior crural nerve.

solution injected while still advancing 1 centimeter deeper. The patient should show some muscular contraction in the thigh, proving that the crural nerve has been reached. The quadriceps is then immediately paralyzed.

Infiltration of the above two nerves affords a broad zone of anesthesia which will permit of the taking of Thiersch grafts from an extensive surface of skin.

Infiltration of the *great sciatic nerve* is very difficult and uncertain. One may, however, succeed in the following manner: Bearing in mind that the nerve is situated in the buttock at the midpoint of a line passing from the ischium to the great trochanter, two deep injections are made, the first at a distance of 2 centimeters outside of the tuberosity of the ischium, and the other 3 centimeters within the great trochanter. Or, a single injection may be made at the intersection of a horizontal line passing through the upper border of the great trochanter, and a vertical line passing through the external border of the ischium. It is indispensable that the patient should experience a painful sensation in the toes. As soon as this pain is felt 10 mils of the strong solution are injected.

Babitzki proceeds as follows: The finger is introduced in the rectum, the lower border of the great sciatic notch identified, and its contents, *i.e.,* the nerve, pushed outward while the right hand introduces the needle to meet the nerve.

The *lesser sciatic nerve* passes below the gluteal fold exactly in the middle of the posterior surface of the thigh, immediately beneath the fascia. It is, therefore, easily accessible.

The *obturator nerve* is deeply situated. To reach it with any degree of certainty all of the proximal internal surface of the thigh should be infiltrated to a depth of 3 or 4 centimeters.

In operating on the great trochanter or the neck of the femur, desensitization of the nerve trunks of the lower extremity is not sufficient; one must also anesthetize the branches of the genito-crural and ilio-inguinal by infiltration of the skin surrounding the root of the extremity.

Operations upon the Toes.

The technique is the same as for the fingers (Figs. 208 and 209). In the case of the big toe, three injections are made, two on the lateral surfaces and one in the middle of the dorsal surface.

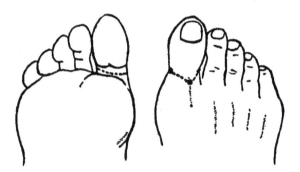

Fig. 207.—Anesthesia of a toe through three dorsal injections. (*Pauchet.*)

A *subcutaneous* ring-shaped injection is made at the root of the member, and 4 or 5 mils of the strong solution injected. For the other toes, the injections are made in the interdigital spaces (Fig. 209).

Great Toe—Operations for Ingrowing Toe Nail or Bunion, Amputation.—In disarticulation of the toe or resection of the head of its metatarsal bone for hallux valgus, three wheals are made, one on the internal border of the foot, the second a dorsal one, above the first interosseous space, and the third in the first interdigital space. One injects

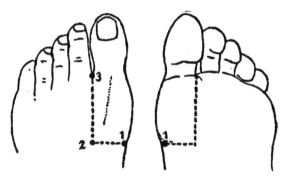

Fig. 208.—Anesthesia of the great toe with the head of its metatarsal bone. (*Pauchet.*)

in the interosseous space, as for the hand. The needle is inserted in this space until its tip touches the deep portion of the skin of the sole. Infiltration is then conducted under the skin from 1 to

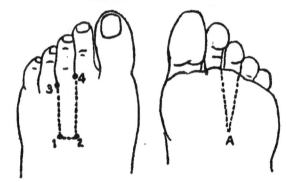

Fig. 209.—Anesthesia of middle toe with the head of its metatarsal bone. (*Pauchet.*)

3, following the dotted line (Fig. 208). Fifty mils of the weak solution are needed.

Third Toe.—Operations on the metatarsal (Fig. 209).—Four wheals are made as in operations

upon the hand—two on the dorsal surface of the
interdigital spaces, and two on the dorsum of the
foot above the second and third interosseous spaces.
Through 1 and 2, anesthetic solution is injected
in the interosseous space until the point of the
needle is perceived under the skin of the sole,
then the injection is continued under the skin of
the dorsum toward 1 and 2. Fifty mils of the
weak solution are required.

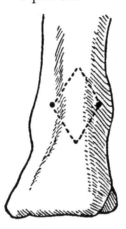

Fig. 210.—Tenotomy of the tendo Achillis. (*Pauchet.*)

TENOTOMY OF THE TENDO ACHILLIS.

A wheal is made on each side, a subcutaneous
diamond formed as shown by the dotted lines in
the illustration (Fig. 210), then infiltration praetised under the tendon itself.

OPERATIONS UPON THE ENTIRE FOOT.

The foot is supplied by five trunks: The anterior and posterior tibial, the internal and external saphenous, and the musculo-cutaneous (Fig.

211). The posterior tibial nerve is injected at the inner malleolus, 1 centimeter from the tendo Achillis (Fig. 211; note the direction of the needle.). The needle is introduced from behind forward up to the posterior surface of the tibia.

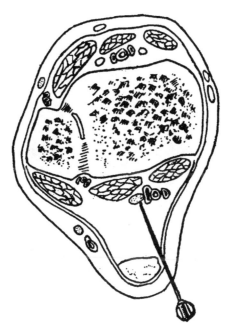

Fig. 211.—Nerves to be infiltrated in anesthetizing the entire foot. (*Pauchet.*) Section of left leg above the malleoli. For the anterior and posterior tibial a deep injection is necessary, and a subcutaneous bracelet for the other nerves, viz., the external and internal saphenous and the musculo-cutaneous.

The operator feels his way until he produces a lancinating pain, and then injects 5 mils of the strong solution. The other wheals are made at the same level around the leg. A subcutaneous bracelet is infiltrated, using 50 to 75 mils of the weak solution, and the strong solution injected to

18

block the anterior tibial, along the line for ligation of the artery of the same name. The resulting anesthesia is sufficient for resections and amputations in the infant and adult (Fig. 212).

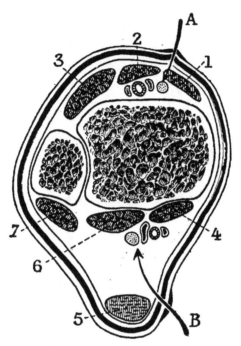

Fig. 212.—Anesthesia of the entire foot. (*Pauchet.*) Horizontal section of left leg above the malleoli. 1, Tibialis anterior. 2, Extensor proprius hallucis. 3, Extensor communis digitorum. 4, Tibialis posterior. 5, Tendo Achillis. 6, Flexor proprius hallucis. 7, Lateral peronei. The black band represents a bracelet of subcutaneous infiltration. *A*, Deep injection for the anterior tibial nerve. *B*, Deep injection for the posterior tibial nerve.

OPERATIONS UPON THE KNEE.

For a hygroma of the prepatellar bursa, four wheals are made (Fig. 213), and the subcutaneous cellular tissue in the interval then infiltrated.

This procedure is also adapted for the suture of a fractured patella. The prepatellar fibrous tissues and the articular cavity itself are infiltrated in. the same way with the strong solution. In suture of the patella, however, 150 to 200 mils of the weak solution are used; the greater part of the solution runs out after the incision.

For foreign body in the knee, the foreign body is first located with the fingers. Then, through a

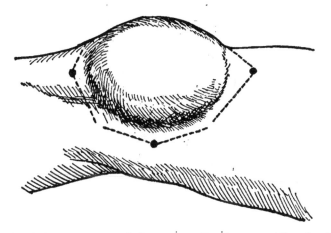

Fig. 213.—Removal of the prepatellar bursa. (*Pauchet.*)

dermal wheal, a needle is introduced, followed by two or three more, to immobilize the foreign body. The skin overlying it is now infiltrated, the fascia likewise, an incision made, the foreign body removed, and the wound sutured. The operation is brilliant, rapid, and painless.

By the same procedure a transverse arthrotomy, with section of the ligamentum patellæ and the lateral ligaments, can very readily be performed. We have in this way removed projec-

tiles embedded in the femoral condyles. Resection
of the condyles can also be done in this way
where the subject is not too stout; but for this
operation we prefer spinal anesthesia. The weak
solution suffices in all cases.

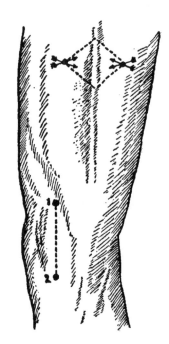

Fig. 214.—Infiltration of a mass of tissue for arthrotomy
of the knee, 1 and 2. (*Pauchet.*) Above, anesthesia of a segment of vein.

OSTEOTOMY OF THE FEMUR.

Supracondylar and subtrochanteric osteotomies
may be practised under local anesthesia by infiltration. On the outer surface of the thigh, at
a height of 10 centimeters, a subcutaneous and
then a subfascial band is traced. Next the muscular mass is infiltrated, down to the bone. Fin-

ally and still by the same route, a long needle is
introduced in front of and outside of the bone,
and the tissues freely infiltrated. The resulting
anesthesia is perfect, the only steps in the operation that are disturbing to the patient being the
breaking of the femur or the blows of the mallet.
The same difficulty is experienced in all bone op-

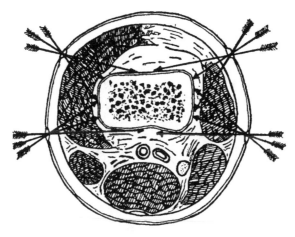

Fig. 215.—Section of the thigh through its lower fourth.
(*Pauchet.*) Manner in which the injections should be directed
for an osteotomy of the femur.

erations. Section of a rib or the removal of a
cranial flap are alike painless manipulations, but
the patient must be warned beforehand of the
sounds caused by section of bone tissue.

OPERATIONS UPON THE SOFT PARTS OF THE THIGH.

The subcutaneous cellular tissues above the
lesion are infiltrated in order to block the subcutaneous nerves. Next, one infiltrates in front

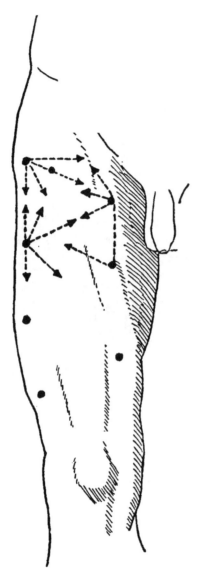

Fig. 216.—Extensive subcutaneous infiltration through
a series of wheals. (*Pauchet.*)

and behind, and when necessary, below. This
constitutes our routine practice for operations on
varicose veins or for inguinal lymphatic enlarge-
ments (see Figs. 216 and 217). The operation
succeeds very well, but a large amount of the

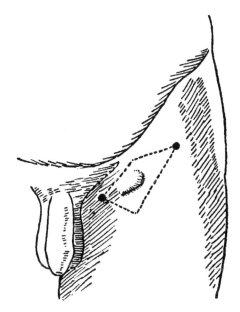

Fig. 217.—Peripheral infiltration of an inguinal lymph-
node for adenitis. (*Pauchet.*)

weak solution is required; this entails no danger,
for a large portion of the solution runs out
through the incision. In the removal of varicose
veins we have commonly used 200, 250, and even
300 grams of the weak solution, which is largely
eliminated when the wound is irrigated with hot
saline solution.

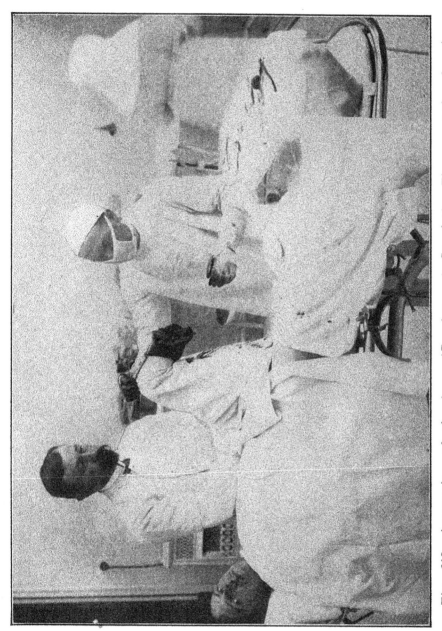

Fig. 218.—Amputation of the leg. (*Pauchet* and *Sourdat*.) The amputation has been carried out after infiltration of the trunks of the anterior crural, great sciatic, and external cutaneous nerves.

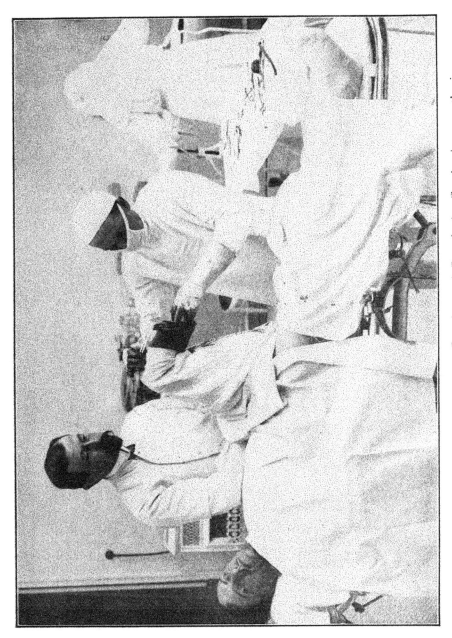

Fig. 219.—Amputation of the leg. (*Pauchet* and *Sourdat*.) Conduction anesthesia.

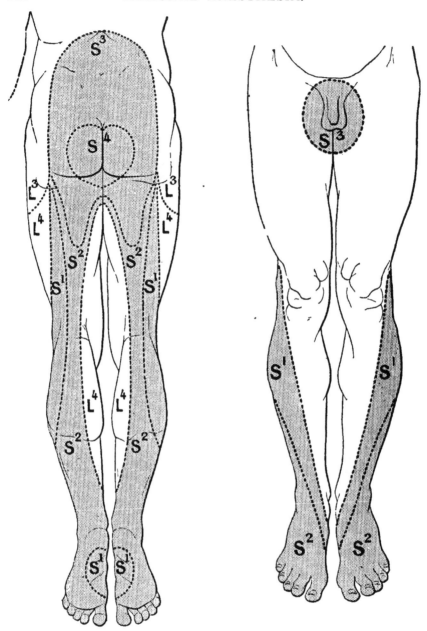

Figs. 220, 221.—Sacral anesthesia of the lower extremity. (*Pauchet.*) The sacral trunks, 1 to 4, require to be injected if one is to obtain the areas of anesthesia shown in the sections *S*. Sections *L3* and *L4* show the anesthesia obtained by paralumbar injection. Sacral anesthesia of the genital organs is conducted through the third foramen. The skin is anesthetized. The reader will note the numbers of the sacral trunks that must be injected to obtain the desired anesthesia.

CONCLUSIONS.[1]

Regional anesthesia may be availed of in 80 per cent. of surgical operations. Its success depends upon the ability and experience of the operator, but the disposition and mental attitude of the patient also play an important part.

We invite beginners to use it not only in one type of case, but systematically in all cases, holding themselves in readiness to use ethyl chloride to, complete the work where necessary.

Cranial nerve anesthesia and the paravertebral, brachial plexus, and trans-sacral procedures, which are most efficacious, require actual training. If our advice to learners is followed, this should not take a long time. Take a hat pin and a skeleton and practice introduction into the cranial foramina, as well as into the paravertebral and sacral openings, in accordance with the landmarks mentioned in this book. Such practice will require one or two hours. The same experimentation should then be carried out upon a cadaver. This will also require about two hours of practice.

After these two series of experiments, trials may be made upon the living subject.

For the remaining operations, trials should be

---

[1] Pauchet-Sourdat-Labouré: Anesthésie régionale—Doin, publisher, Paris, 1917.

made with the book by one's side, as is done by the internes in my service.

Be gentle, patient, and persevering in spite of failures and the aversion of certain patients, and you will succeed, with signal benefit to most cases and with general advancement of surgical practice.

INDEX.

(285)

CPSIA information can be obtained
at www.ICGtesting.com
Printed in the USA
BVHW03*0633290518
517623BV00012B/27/P

9 780364 440872